Antidepressants and the Pharmaceutical Companies

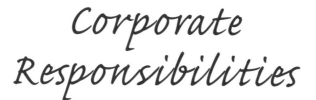

Corporate Responsibilities

ANTIDEPRESSANTS

ANTIDEPRESSANTS

Antidepressants and the Pharmaceutical Companies

Corporate Responsibilities

by David Hunter

Mason Crest Publishers

Philadelphia

Mason Crest Publishers Inc.
370 Reed Road
Broomall, Pennsylvania 19008
(866) MCP-BOOK (toll free)

First printing
1 2 3 4 5 6 7 8 9 10
Library of Congress Cataloging-in-Publication Data

Hunter, David.
  Antidepressants and the pharmaceutical companies : corporate responsi-
bilities / by David Hunter.
      p. cm. — (Antidepressants)
  Includes bibliographical references and index.
  ISBN 1-4222-0101-5   ISBN 1-4222-0094-9 (series)
  1. Antidepressants—Juvenile literature. 2. Pharmaceutical industry—
Juvenile literature. I. Title. II. Series.
  RM332.H863 2007
  615'.78—dc22
                              2006005486

Interior design by MK Bassett-Harvey.
Interiors produced by Harding House Publishing Service, Inc.
www.hardinghousepages.com.
Cover design by Peter Culatta.
Printed in the Hashemite Kingdom of Jordan.

This book is meant to educate and should not be used as an alternative to appropriate medical care. Its creators have made every effort to ensure that the information presented is accurate—but it is not intended to substitute for the help and
services of trained professionals.

Contents

Introduction

by Andrew M. Kleiman, M.D.

From ancient Greece through the twenty-first century, the experience of sadness and depression is one of the many that define humanity. As long as human beings have felt emotions, they have endured depression. Experienced by people from every race, socioeconomic class, age group, and culture, depression is an emotional and physical experience that millions of people suffer each day. Despite being described in literature and music; examined by countless scientists, philosophers, and thinkers; and studied and treated for centuries, depression continues to remain as complex and mysterious as ever.

In today's Western culture, hearing about depression and treatments for depression is common. Adolescents in particular are bombarded with information, warnings, recommendations, and suggestions. It is critical that adolescents and young people have an understanding of depression and its impact on an individual's psychological and physical health, as well as the treatment options available to help those who suffer from depression.

Why? Because depression can lead to poor school performance, isolation from family and friends, alcohol and drug abuse, and even suicide. This doesn't have to be the case, since many useful and promising treatments exist to relieve the suffering of those with depression. Treatments for depression may also pose certain risks, however.

Since the beginning of civilization, people have been trying to alleviate the suffering of those with depression. Modern-day medicine and psychology have taken the understanding and treatment of depression to new heights. Despite their shortcomings, these treatments have helped millions and millions of people lead happier, more fulfilling and prosperous lives that would not be possible in generations past. These treatments, however, have their own risks, and for some people, may not be effective at all. Much work in neuroscience, medicine, and psychology needs to be done in the years to come.

Many adolescents experience depression, and this book series will help young people to recognize depression both in themselves and in those around them. It will give them the basic understanding of the history of depression and the various treatments that have been used to combat depression over the years. The books will also provide a basic scientific understanding of depression, and the many biological, psychological, and alternative treatments available to someone suffering from depression today.

Each person's brain and biology, life experiences, thoughts, and day-to-day situations are unique. Similarly, each individual experiences depression and sadness in a unique way. Each adolescent suffering from depression thus requires a distinct, individual treatment plan that best suits his or her needs. This series promises to be a vital resource for helping young people recognize and understand depression, and make informed and thoughtful decisions regarding treatment.

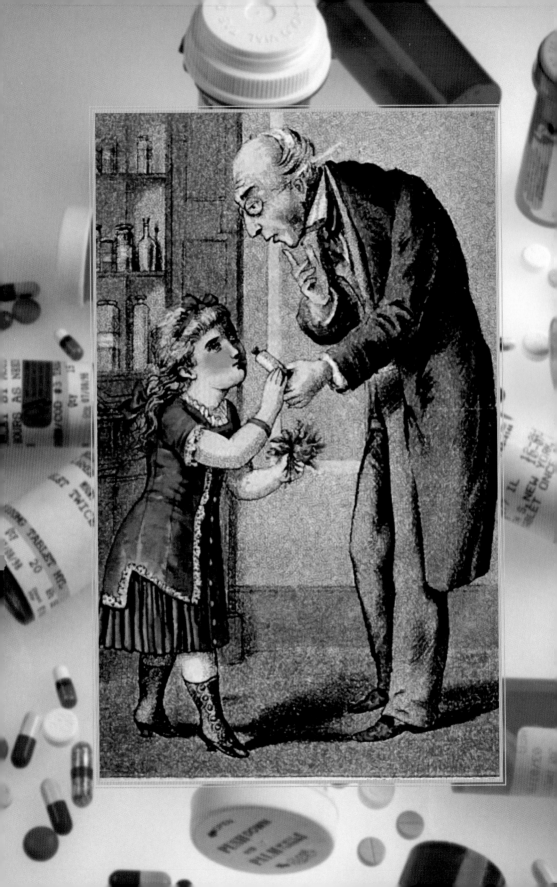

Chapter 1

The Growth of the Pharmaceutical Industry

When we take medicines, we don't generally stop to think about how those medicines are discovered and developed. Nor do we think much about the business behind that medicine—the money involved in producing the medicine, the revenues earned from sales of the medicine, and the governmental agencies that regulate the development and marketing of drugs. In general, most people are only concerned that the medicines they take make them feel better.

That most of the drugs we use do work when we take them is a testament to the effectiveness of the processes and agencies involved in drug development. That's not to say that there aren't problems in the system, however. The pharmaceutical industry has its fair share of successes, failures, and controversies. In fact, every drug has a story behind it. In the case of antidepressants in particular, those stories can be quite complicated and often highly **controversial**.

The pharmaceutical industry has done a great deal of good for the world, bringing us cures for many deadly sicknesses, drugs that help alleviate pain and suffering, and even medicines that help to improve psychological conditions such as depression. The industry's enormous profits and growth in the past century, however, and most particularly in the last two decades, have caused some people to grow suspicious of its motivations. With success has come criticism and **skepticism**.

Perhaps it's a bit unfair to say that criticism and skepticism have come only with success. In fact, looking back at the history of the pharmaceutical industry, we can see that it has always had its share of critics.

The Early Pharmaceutical Industry

Since the first recorded history, and undoubtedly well before that, people have made use of both plant and animal parts as medicines. Many ancient civilizations had complicated medical theories that fostered the use of these materials. While some of these medicinal mixtures worked, others proved to be fairly ineffective in treating the conditions for which they were created. In some cases, the medicines were actually toxic, making them more deadly than the illnesses they treated.

Some old medicines and folk remedies, however, have continued to be used even today. St. John's wort, for example, was used in ancient Greece for a variety of purposes. It was applied to wounds to help them heal faster and to rid the body of infections. Most notably, it was used to treat what were once known as "nervous conditions," which we now understand as depression, and a variety of other psychological disorders. St. John's wort is still one of the most commonly used herbal remedies in the treatment of mild or moderate depression.

As late as the beginning of the twentieth century, medicine was more of an art than a science. In fact, many medicines seemed to rely more on **theatrics** and creative marketing than on proof of effectiveness. Medicines carried names that encouraged people to buy them and use them—catchy names like "Kick-a-poo Indian Sagwa" or reassuring, descriptive names such as "Warner's Safe Cure for Diabetes." What's more, sales of many medicines involved a great deal of

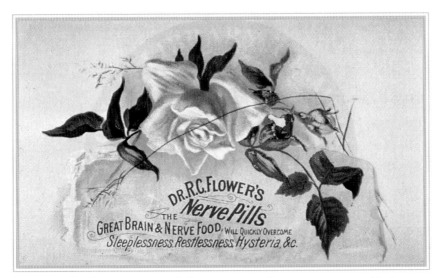

At the beginning of the twentieth century, medicine advertisements made extravagant claims and encouraged buyers to associate their products with health, beauty, and family values.

showmanship. Salesmen touting Hamlin's Wizard Oil, for instance, traveled with a **veritable** circus act of entertainers and animals. Their purpose was to draw attention to the product they sold—and sell it they did. Such shows were a common sight in nineteenth-century North American towns.

Unfortunately, pomp and bravado are not guarantees of effectiveness. In fact, most of the medicines available in the nineteenth and early twentieth centuries were ineffective. Even the best-selling medicine of the nineteenth century, Lydia Pinkham's Vegetable Compound, was financially successful not because it worked, but rather, because it was a trusted name brand. Scientific analysis of the compound showed that it was 20 percent alcohol, with the remainder being a variety of vegetable **extracts**. Drinking a glass of fruit or vegetable juice would be just as effective as this medication, and better for you to boot.

Still, some medicines that were developed in the nineteenth century did hold some verifiable medicinal value. Some of these medicines are still used by doctors, hospitals, and general consumers. Aspirin, for instance, was developed in the late nineteenth century and is still commonly used for pain relief, to reduce fevers, and to prevent heart attacks. The vaccines for **diphtheria** and **tetanus** were also discovered in the nineteenth century and are still important today.

Prior to 1906, anybody with a recipe for a cure, a bit of **charisma**, and the motivation to make some money could sell concoctions and call them medicine. To a large extent, the pharmaceutical industry was ruled by the profit motive,

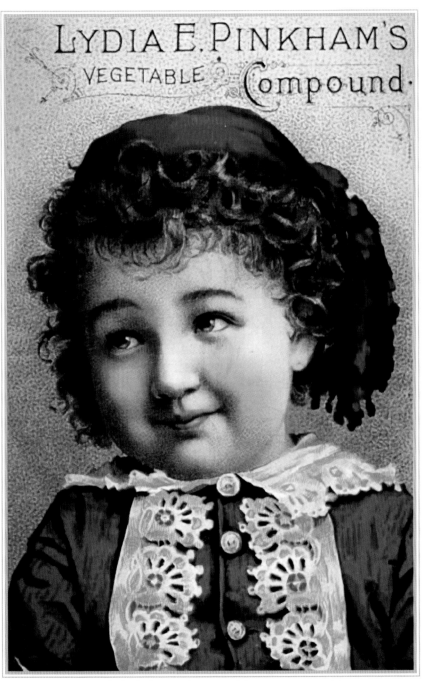

The label for Lydia Pinkham's Vegetable Compound inspired consumers' trust.

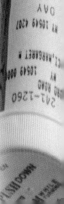

and salesmen peddled hopes rather than cures. It was in this atmosphere that the pharmaceutical industry had its start. Fortunately, the effectiveness of genuine drugs slowly became apparent, and in time those companies that made ineffective products failed. As more **potent** medicines became available and more money was spent on advertising them, expenditures on drugs rose dramatically.

In 1859, just prior to the American Civil War, sales of manufactured medicines reached about 3.5 million dollars per year. By 1904, sales of manufactured medicines had risen to almost 75 million dollars per year. By comparison, at the height of its sales in the late 1990s, a single blockbuster drug—Prozac® (fluoxetine hydrochloride)—netted as much in less than two weeks of sales. Today, the North American pharmaceutical industry is huge, with annual sales of prescription drugs topping 200 billion dollars in 2002.

Although the science behind drug development and the technology behind the manufacture of drugs have continued to progress throughout the history of the pharmaceutical industry, it was not until World War II that the pace of development truly leapt forward. World War II created a tremendous demand for new, more effective medical compounds, largely to treat injured and sick soldiers. After World War II, as industry and science turned their efforts away from wartime research and development and back toward more peaceful pursuits, the pharmaceutical industry entered a period of explosive growth and development that has continued to this day. During this time of rapid scientific breakthroughs, the first modern antidepressant medications were created.

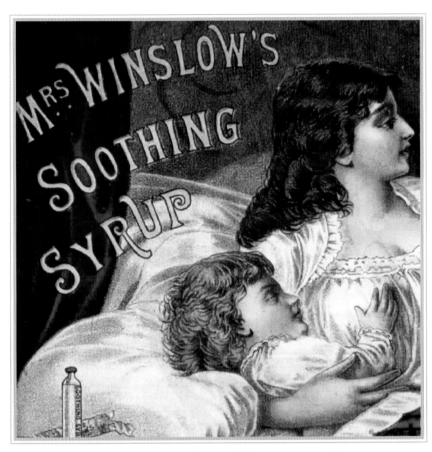

In the 1880s, products like Mrs. Winslow's Soothing Syrup helped increase the sales of manufactured medicines in the United States.

The Development of Antidepressants

As we have already seen, herbal remedies for nervous conditions have long been a component of folk and herbal medicine. The first commercial drug used as an antidepressant, however, may well be Dr. A. W. Chase's Nervous Pills (known as Dr. Chase's Nervous Food in Canada), a brand of medicine that

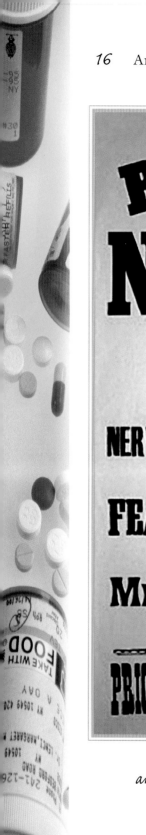

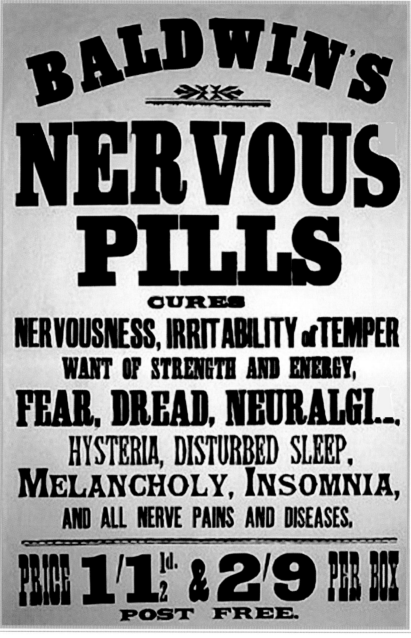

While Dr. Chase promised to cure America's and Canada's nervous complaints, Dr. Baldwin made similar promises in England.

was popular during the late nineteenth and early twentieth centuries. Dr. Chase's Nervous Pills were widely advertised in newspapers during the time and became a popular remedy for nervous conditions.

In the early twentieth century, when Dr. Chase's Nervous Pills were popular, depression was recognized by medical professionals, but not in the same way that it is recognized today. In general, medical disorders were considered at that time to be a weakening of some function of the body. In the case of depression, it was seen as a weakening of the nerves. In fact, most psychological conditions were referred to under the blanket term of "weak nerves." Some doctors also referred to these conditions as "neurasthenia," but this diagnosis was so broad that, by today's standards, it was really not a very useful categorization. Whether a person was suffering from what we now understand to be depression, ***obsessive-compulsive disorder***, or an anxiety disorder, doctors at the beginning of the twentieth century called it weak nerves or neurasthenia.

According to one newspaper advertisement in the *Newark Advocate* from December 6, 1904, Dr. Chase's Nervous Pills were "the natural and rational way to restore the wasted and exhausted nerves." This sort of rationale behind the use and effects of the medicine was common in the early days of pharmaceuticals. It highlights the notion that an effective medication is one that restores and revitalizes the natural function of the body. Today, we understand that illness is generally much more complicated than that, and effective medicines work by targeting various chemical processes that occur in the body.

This understanding of disease and medical treatment gained ground quickly in the first half of the twentieth century, but technology and science lacked the sophistication to pinpoint the exact processes that governed disease and recovery. Nevertheless, through a great deal of trial-and-error experimentation, observation, and perhaps a bit of luck, the post–World War II years saw a great deal of innovation in drug development.

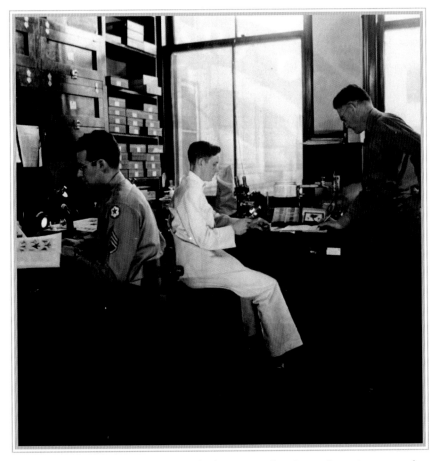

World War II stimulated the growth of medical research.

Brand Name vs. Generic Name

Talking about psychiatric drugs can be confusing, because every drug has at least two names: its "generic name" and the "brand name" that the pharmaceutical company uses to market the drug. Generic names come from the drugs' chemical structure, while drug companies use brand names in order to inspire public recognition and loyalty for their products.

In the 1950s, researchers stumbled on several chemical compounds that appeared to be successful in the treatment of depression. One of these, Marsilid® (iproniazid), was categorized as a monoamine oxidase inhibitor (MAOI). This rather long name described how the medicine worked, namely by inhibiting a chemical process in the brain. Marsilid itself was described as a "psychic energizer," because it tended to give people increased energy. This description of Marsilid gives a good indication that the scientific understanding of depression was still not very advanced at the time this drug was developed. Indeed, the term "psychic energizer" echoes the language used to describe Dr. Chase's Nervous Pills fifty years before. Although Marsilid seemed effective in treating depression, a host of side effects made it unsafe for many people to use. It was removed from the market after a very short time.

Another antidepressant that was introduced at around the same time was marketed under the name Tofranil® (imipramine hydrochloride). Tofranil was the first tricyclic antidepressant, so named for its three-ring chemical structure. Like Marsilid, Tofranil appeared to be effective in the treatment of depression. Unlike Marsilid, it had a **sedative** effect rather than a **stimulant** effect. That both drugs could effectively be used in the treatment of depression raised many questions among researchers interested in the mechanisms that caused depression. How, after all, could a sedative relieve depression if a stimulant did too?

It became very clear to researchers that they did not understand the chemistry or the causes of depression. Nevertheless, other tricyclic and MAOI drugs followed. If not for the fact that all of them had a long list of uncomfortable and sometimes potentially dangerous side effects, the development of other antidepressants might not have occurred. As it was, however, few doctors would prescribe these early antidepressants except in the most serious cases of depression. The risks of taking the medicines were simply too high to justify the possible benefits.

More than two more decades would pass before that would finally change. In 1987, a drug was introduced that changed the way that doctors and patients related to depression. That drug was Prozac (fluoxetine hydrochloride), produced by pharmaceutical company Eli Lilly. More than almost any other drug, Prozac marked a turning point for the pharmaceutical industry, for health care, and for patients.

Prozac was the first of a new class of antidepressants called selective serotonin reuptake inhibitors, or SSRIs. Unlike the earlier MAOIs and tricyclics, the SSRI class of drugs carries with it few side effects. At the time Prozac was introduced, in fact, it appeared to have almost no serious side effects at all. Doctors and psychiatrists could feel much more comfortable prescribing it to patients with mild or moderate

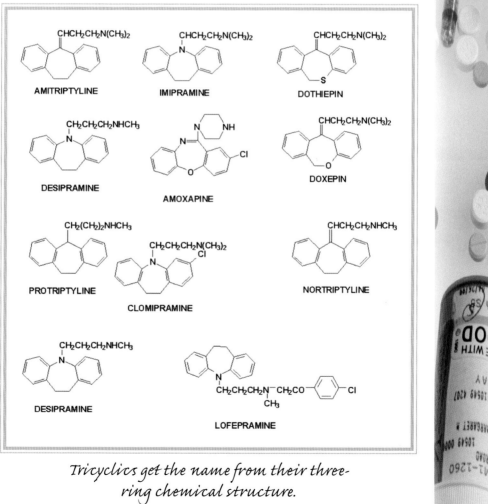

Tricyclics get the name from their three-ring chemical structure.

depression—patients who would not have received treatment with the more problematic MAOIs and tricyclics.

Other SSRIs soon followed Prozac onto the market. In 1992, Paxil® (paroxetine hydrochloride) and Zoloft® (sertraline hydrochloride) entered the market. Luvox® (fluvoxamine maleate) joined the race in 1995, followed by Celexa® (citalopram hydrobromide) in 1998 and then Lexapro® (escitalopram oxalate), a derivative of Celexa, in 2002. As a whole, the SSRIs have been one of the most successful classes of drugs ever sold. Another type of antidepressant—serotonin and norepinephrine reuptake inhibitors, or SNRIs—has also enjoyed a good deal of financial success, though not to the extent of the SSRIs.

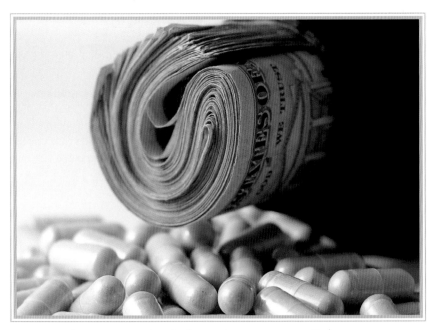

Pharmaceuticals have become one of the most profitable industries in the world.

Sales of SSRIs and SNRIs have helped the antidepressant class of drugs become one of the most profitable classes of drugs in North America. In 2002, antidepressants ranked third in overall sales of prescription medicines in the United States, earning a whopping 17.1 billion dollars. Paxil and Zoloft were both ranked among the top-ten individual drugs sold for that year; sales of Paxil totaled 3.3 billion dollars and those of Zoloft totaled 2.9 billion dollars. What's more, sales of these drugs and other antidepressants have been rising rapidly every year. Between 2000 and 2001, in fact, sales of antidepressants rose faster than sales of any other drug class.

Contrary to what the rapid rise in antidepressant sales over the past decade would seem to indicate, many critics contend that the drugs are not as effective as the pharmaceutical companies claim they are. This criticism is directed not only at the drug companies that produce the medicines, but also at the governments that allow them to be produced and marketed.

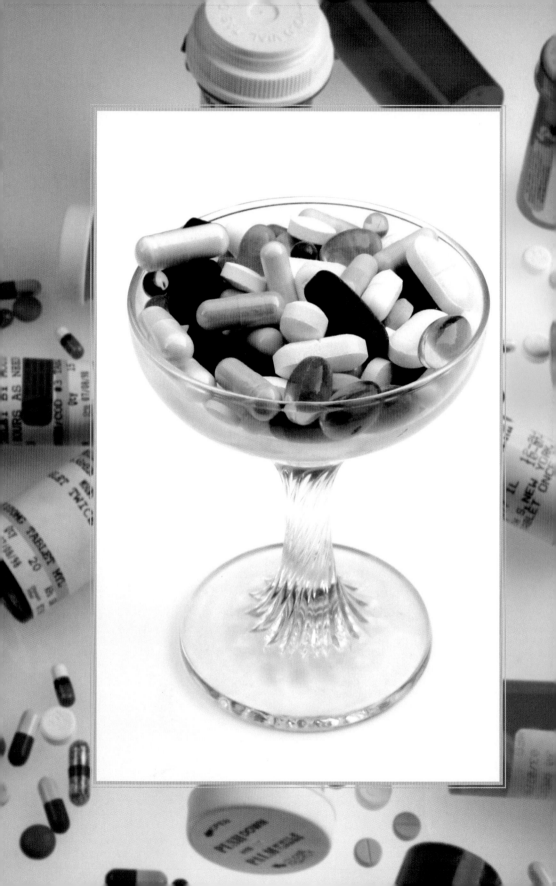

Chapter 2

Regulation: The Development of the FDA

*T*he history and rise of government agencies—such as Health Canada and the FDA, the United States' Food and Drug Administration—have been closely intertwined with the history and growth of the pharmaceutical industry has been. These organizations were founded to help safeguard the health of people living in these countries by regulating North Americans' food, as well as the growing pharmaceutical industry. Both the FDA and Health Canada were given the responsibility of ensuring that the drugs produced by pharmaceutical companies meet certain standards of effectiveness and safety. Not surprisingly, these agencies had their origins in the early twentieth century, when uncertainty over pharmaceutical products was rampant and the safety of many medicines was in question.

Almost on Target: The Origins of the FDA

In 1906, the Congress of the United States passed the Pure Food and Drug Act. This new law aimed to reduce misin-

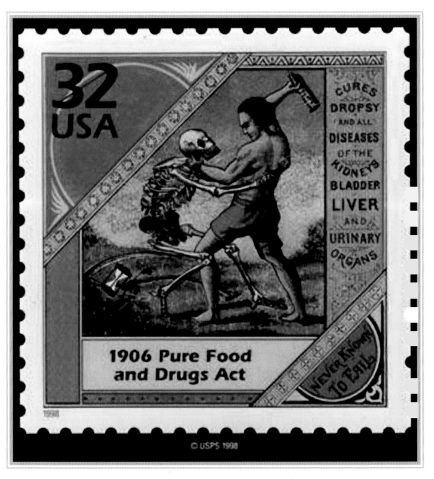

The U.S. Postal Service issued this stamp in 1998 to commemorate the passage of the Pure Food and Drug Act in 1906.

formation regarding drugs sold in the country and to limit the number of dangerous foods and medicines on the market. First and foremost, it prohibited the manufacture and sale of drugs that were poisonous. In addition, it required manufacturers to list on their product labels any dangerous or addictive ingredients in those products and prohibited the sale of medicines and foods that were mislabeled or misbranded—which, for the most part, meant products with inaccurate or false ingredient listings.

At the time, all these issues were major concerns for consumers because many medicines contained ingredients that were more harmful than helpful, including alcohol, cocaine, and opium. While the legislation was an important step toward reining in the chaotic pharmaceutical industry, it fell short of being a truly effective regulatory measure.

In hindsight, the Pure Food and Drug Act had several major flaws. For one, the law did not prohibit narcotic ingredients and alcohol as ingredients in medicines; it only required that addictive and dangerous ingredients of that nature be listed on the labels of any medicines in which they were a component. It did not, however, require any indication of the amount of these ingredients. Nor did the law address the many fake and useless concoctions that people sold as medicines.

The Sherley Amendment of 1912 addressed this last problem by requiring that any therapeutic claims made about a medicine be valid and true. According to the new amendment, any company that made false claims about the range of medical conditions a drug could treat or about the effectiveness of that drug in treating those conditions could be taken to court over the issue. The courts could then force any companies in violation of the law to pay fines to the government and to change their claims about the therapeutic value of the drug.

Like the original Pure Food and Drug Act that it modified, however, the Sherley Amendment failed to produce results in a key way. The lawmakers who had drafted the new amendment had placed the burden of proving such claims to be false on the government. Unfortunately, the government lacked the resources to pursue violators of the amendment, and many of those they did take to court were able to escape legal action. The science of the time was simply not sophisticated enough to prove that many questionable drugs were ineffective. Though the Sherley Amendment had been a step in the right direction for government regulation of the pharmaceutical industry, it lacked the teeth to make a significant impact.

One difficulty in this regard was the lack of a government agency dedicated to the regulation of the pharmaceutical industry. At the time the Sherley Amendment was drafted, regulatory powers rested with the Bureau of Chemistry. The Bureau of Chemistry, however, was not merely a **regulatory agency** but also had research and development responsibilities. As the number of medicines on the market continued to rise, the task of ensuring the safety and **efficacy** of those medicines became increasingly difficult. Due to its other involvements and responsibilities, the resources of the Bureau of Chemistry were simply inadequate for the task.

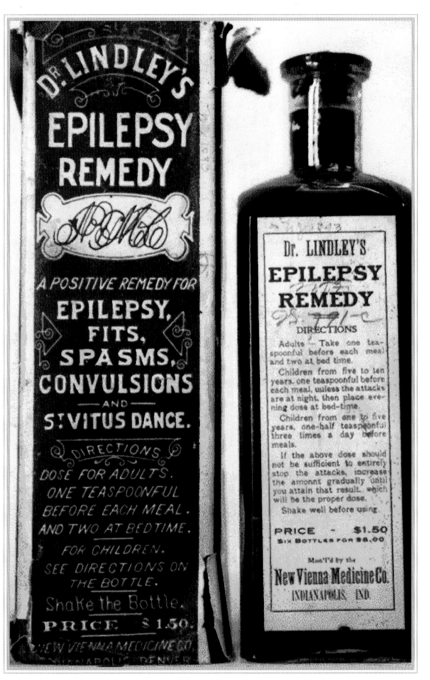

A governmental agency was needed to regulate the claims made by medicinal products like this one.

CERTIFICATE OF PURITY

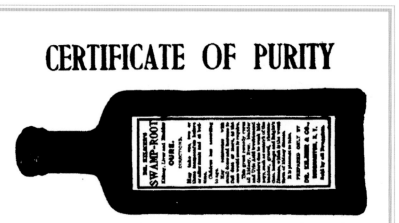

This is to Certify that Dr. Kilmer's Swamp-Root, the great kidney, liver and bladder remedy, is purely vegetable and does not contain any calomel, mercury, creosote, morphine, opium, strychnine, cocaine, nitrate potash (salt-petre), bromide potassium, narcotic alkaloid, whiskey, wine or any harmful or habit producing drugs. Swamp-Root was discovered through scientific research and study by Dr. Kilmer, who graduated with honors and is now actively engaged in the practice of his profession, which calling he has successfully followed many years.   State of New York, County of Broome, } S. S.
City of Binghamton,

Jonas M. Kilmer, senior member of the firm of Dr. Kilmer & Co., of the City of Binghamton, County of Broome, State of New York, being duly sworn, deposes and says that the guarantee of purity of Swamp-Root, as described in the foregoing certificate, is in all respects true.

Subscribed and sworn to
before me April 26. 1898.

Jonas M. Kilmer

Dr. Kilmer's **Swamp-Root** is not recommended for everything, but if you have kidney, liver or bladder trouble, it will be found just the remedy you need. Swamp-Root makes friends.
Each bottle contains the same standard of purity, strength and excellence.
You may have a sample bottle of Swamp-Root free by mail, if you have not already had one.
When writing to Dr. Kilmer & Co., Binghamton, N. Y., be sure to mention reading this generous offer in this paper.
If you are already convinced that Swamp-Root is what you need, you can purchase the regular fifty cent and one-dollar size bottles at drug stores everywhere. Don't make any mistake, but remember the name, Swamp-Root, Dr. Kilmer's Swamp-Root, and the address, Binghamton N. Y. on every bottle.

Although Dr. Kilmer told buyers that his Swamp-Root was "pure," the passage of the Food, Drug, and Cosmetic Act meant that such drug companies as Dr. Kilmer's had to prove their claims to the government.

In 1927, the Bureau of Chemistry was divided into two distinct groups: the Bureau of Chemistry and Soils, which oversaw research, and the Food, Drug, and Insecticide Administration, which oversaw food and drug regulation. In 1931, the Food, Drug, and Insecticide Administration became the Food and Drug Administration. Although the birth of the FDA indicated an increased desire by the federal government to regulate the pharmaceutical industry, the loopholes present in existing drug laws continued to hinder effective regulation.

That situation would finally change in 1938, when Congress passed the Food, Drug, and Cosmetic Act. In essence, the Food, Drug, and Cosmetic Act reiterated the intent of the 1906 and 1912 laws, but it also took them a step further. Rather than requiring the FDA to prove that a drug was safe and effective, the 1938 act placed that responsibility on the company producing the drug, where it still rests today. Furthermore, in order for a drug to be released on the market and sold in the United States, it had to first receive clearance from the FDA. Ostensibly, this clearance would be given on demonstration of the safety and effectiveness of the new drug. Standards and procedures for proving these requirements, however, would not be developed for many years.

Nevertheless, the 1938 law marked a major moment in the development of the FDA. While the laws before it had been important steps in setting the stage for government regulation of the industry, the Food, Drug, and Cosmetic Act set the course for the development of both the modern drug approval process and the fledgling FDA.

Compromises and Controversies: The FDA and the Growth of Big Pharmaceuticals

Further revisions to U.S. drug law would come in 1951 with the passage of the Durham-Humphrey Amendment to the Food, Drug, and Cosmetics Act. This amendment designated drugs that could be habit-forming or toxic as prescription drugs, available only with the approval of a physician. Until then, the drug companies themselves determined which drugs were available by prescription and which were available without prescription. With the Durham-Humphrey Amendment, the FDA asserted its authority, setting a powerful precedent for the future.

Like all the drug laws passed before it, though, the Durham-Humphrey Amendment had mixed results in terms of regulating the pharmaceutical industry. On the one hand, it was clear that **indiscriminate** use of certain drugs posed a serious health threat to people. By requiring physician approval of those drugs, it reduced the number of people inappropriately or dangerously using the medicines, thereby safeguarding people from unnecessary harm. Passage of the amendment, however, also coincided with the rapid rise in new drug development that followed World War II. Because of this, the new law paved the way for unprecedented financial gains by the pharmaceutical industry.

Prior to 1951, few drug varieties were available on the market. Consequently, very few drugs fit the amendment's criteria for classification as prescription drugs. In the 1950s, however,

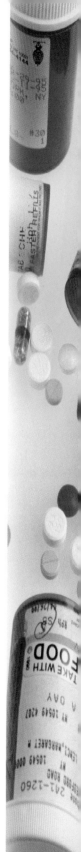

the industry experienced a burst of new drug development. Many of these new drugs fit the amendment's guidelines and could be marketed only as prescription drugs, a categorization that had been relatively uncommon up to that point. For a wide variety of reasons, prescription drugs are, on average, much more expensive than **over-the-counter** nonprescription drugs.

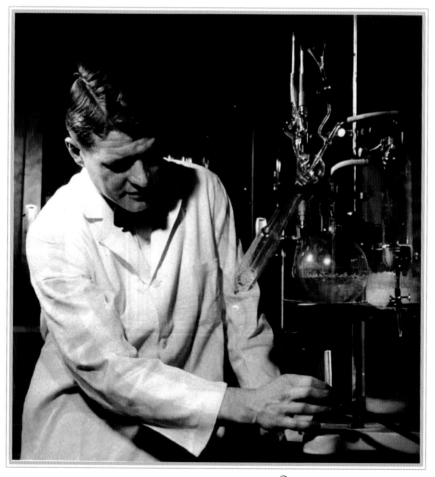

During the 1950s, researchers developed many new drugs.

In fact, brand-name prescription drugs generally cost many times more than over-the-counter nonprescription drugs. For example, in 2003, the FDA switched the popular antihistamine and decongestant Claritin® from prescription to nonprescription status. Before that time, a month supply of Claritin cost about ninety-six dollars. After the switch, brand-name Claritin cost only about twenty-two dollars for a one-month supply. Generic loratadine, the active ingredient in Claritin, can be purchased for as little as ten dollars for a month supply. The new legislation helped to make the pharmaceutical industry one of the most profitable industries in the world.

In 1962, the Kefauver-Harris Amendment was added to the Food, Drug, and Cosmetic Act. This amendment forced drug manufacturers to prove the effectiveness of their prod-

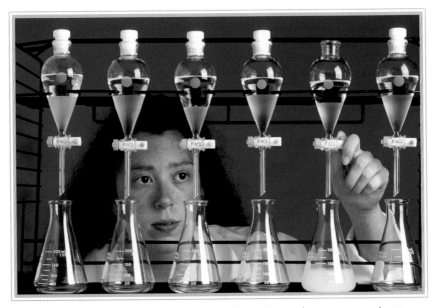

Researchers often work hand in hand with FDA regulations.

ucts before they could be marketed. What's more, the amendment set down guidelines and procedures for establishing drug efficacy. This marked the birth of the modern drug approval process. The Kefauver-Harris Amendment also required pharmaceutical companies to provide comprehensive information about the risks and benefits of their medications in all promotional materials to physicians. At the time, drug companies could not advertise prescription drugs directly to consumers, which made doctors the only source of medical information for many people. By requiring honest appraisals of the risks of certain medication in promotional materials to physicians, the FDA helped to better educate those physicians, and thus better protect the consumer.

In 1997, the FDA relaxed restrictions against direct-to-consumer advertising—commonly known as DTC advertising. Up to that point, companies were heavily restricted in the ways they could promote prescription drugs. Advertisements in medical journals, visits to hospitals and doctors, and the sponsorship of continuing education courses for physicians allowed pharmaceutical companies to promote their products to physicians and other medical professionals. For the most part, however, they could not advertise directly to the general public. Once the FDA lifted the restriction on DTC advertising, pharmaceutical companies began pouring money into advertising in a way they had never done before, and the pharmaceutical industry began to experience unprecedented growth.

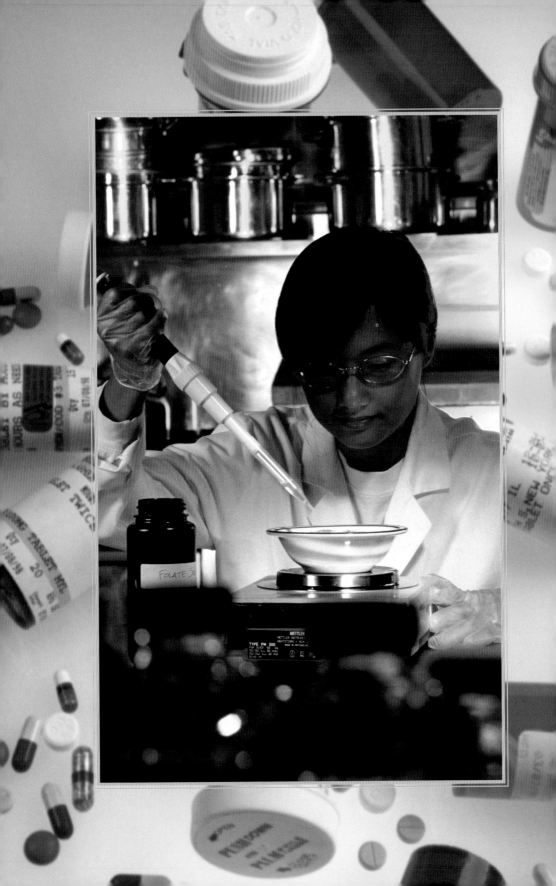

Chapter 3

The Drug Development Process

The story of the drug development process has also been the story of the progress of technology. As pharmaceutical technology and basic understanding of chemistry and biology have evolved, so too has the way in which drugs are developed.

Since humanity first began experimenting with plant and animal compounds as possible remedies for illness, people have been searching for cures to a wide range of conditions. Some of these remedies are questionable, at the very least, while others have proved to be effective.

Browsing through a nutrition store or an organic food and remedies store, you will find a great many different plant compounds such as ginseng, gingko biloba, and kava kava.

Many of these naturally occurring chemicals have scientifically proven effects on the human body, both therapeutic and otherwise. Many others, however, remain unproven. These latter chemicals seem to succeed financially due not to scientific proof of their effectiveness, but rather because of the experiences of the people who use and promote them.

One such chemical is St. John's wort, which grows wild in many parts of Europe and North America. As was already mentioned in chapter 1, many people use St. John's wort today as a natural antidepressant. Studies, however, have been **inconclusive** as to how effective it is in treating depression. Some studies have shown that it is more effective than some standard antidepressant drugs; other studies show that it is no more effective than a placebo (a pill that, unknown to the patient, has no medicinal qualities). Regardless, St. John's wort is available in many places without a prescription, and many people swear by its effectiveness. However, just because a substance is "natural" does not mean that it does not contain chemicals—and these chemicals can affect the body in both good and bad ways; St. John's wort has its own set of side effects and possible interactions with other medications.

In contrast to many of the medicines you can now find in the pharmacy, creating your own medical preparation from a plant such as St. John's wort is fairly simple. Teas, plant extracts, and ground **poultices** of plants are still used in many parts of the world for their purported therapeutic effects, and can be prepared in most kitchens. Even as late as the nineteenth century, in many parts of North America, this was an

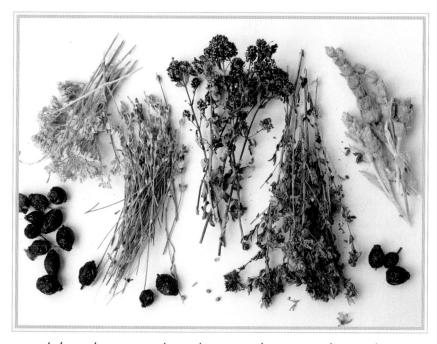

Although "natural medicines" that come from plants are often considered to be safer, these treatments also contain chemicals that can have unwanted side effects.

important way by which people treated themselves medically. As society became more specialized and the pharmaceutical industry more sophisticated, however, people stopped creating their own medications and began buying the more complicated compounds offered by salesmen, pharmacists, and doctors.

In the nineteenth and early twentieth centuries, as we saw, many of the available medicines were little more than empty promises by quack salesmen. In many cases, the manufacturers of these compounds would claim that their medicines

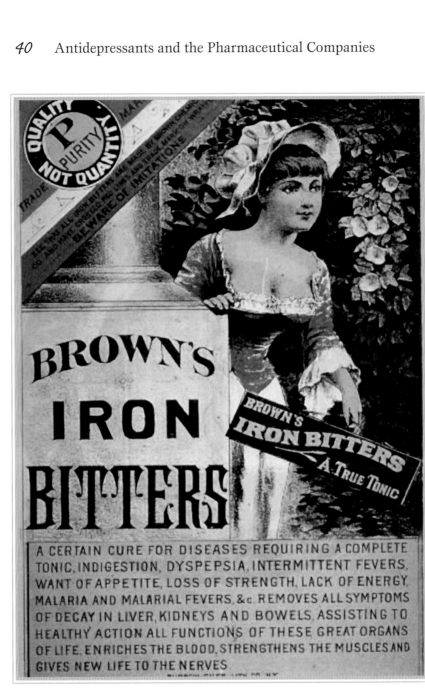

This "tonic" claimed to cure "indigestion, dyspepsia, intermittent fevers, lack of appetite, loss of strength, lack of energy, malaria" and remove "all symptoms of decay in liver, kidneys, and bowels," while enriching the blood, strengthening the muscles, and giving new life to nerves.

could treat a wide variety of conditions. A person might say that a single concoction could treat conditions ranging from an upset stomach to headaches to smelly feet to depression. Unfortunately for the people using these compounds, most of them were not effective in treating any of these conditions, let alone all of them at once.

Fortunately, the establishment of the FDA helped to cut down on such false medications. It was not until the science became available to ensure the safety and efficacy of drugs, however, that quack medicines were eliminated from the market. That same science has played a major role in changing the way that medicines are developed.

Drug Development Before the Regulation Era

Many people think of the nineteenth and early twentieth centuries as a sort of dark age of medicine in North America. While in some places this may be accurate, it is too broad of a generalization to apply everywhere. Indeed, in the cities of North America, some very exciting medical research was being conducted, and the science of medicine was being advanced.

In more rural areas, however, inadequate access to hospitals and pharmacists resulted in many people having no reliable sources of information about drugs, their effectiveness, and their side effects. False drug salesmen thrived for this very reason. Although their claims for the effects of their drugs seem today to be fantastic and *farcical*, to many rural folk of the nineteenth century, the hope **engendered** in those medicines was well worth the expense. Quacks and false drug salesmen profited tidily from the lack of scientific sophistication of the time.

Today, of course, such characters as wandering drug salesmen have long since been relegated to history. Although their medications were generally ineffective, they nevertheless served a valuable role in the development of modern drug research and development, as well as in the growth of the FDA and other regulatory agencies like it. The very uncontrolled nature of these characters and the uncertain nature of their medicines caused the pharmaceutical industry and the government to react, ensuring that scientific validation of therapeutic claims and safety would become standards by which medicines are now developed. In a sense, it was false medicine that led to the development of the FDA and the modern drug development process.

Thorazine®: Precursor to Antidepressants

Despite the intentions of early legislation regarding drug development and marketing, the science and technology necessary to carry out meaningful validation of the safety and effectiveness of drugs was still a long way off. In the early years of the twentieth century, few methods were available to check that a manufacturer's claims about a drug were accurate. What's more, the drug manufacturers themselves had no way to know what the effects of an experimental drug would be until they could observe its effects in test subjects. Such

STIMULATION WITHOUT INTOXICATION.

The boasted nourishing and strengthening properties of Lager Beer, Ale, Porter and other Malt Liquors, and even Malt Extracts, which are nothing but strong Lager Beer, reside solely in the alcohol they contain, which, while temporarily overcoming fatigue and distress, entails upon their devotees the dreaded consumption of the Kidneys and Liver, Dropsy, Piles and Impoverishment of the Blood now so universal. *Fermentation totally destroys the medicinal virtues of Malt by conversion into alcohol.*

BEWARE OF IMITATIONS.

EVERY BOTTLE HOLDS NEALY ONE QUART.

MINIATURE FAC-SIMILIE OF MALT BITTERS.

MALT BITTERS
TRADE MARK

MALT BITTERS

Is prepared without fermentation or the development of alcohol, from Malt, Hops, Quinine Bark, Pyrophosphate Iron, &c., and is the most Nourishing Food ever compounded. It is adapted to the most delicate mother or child, and contains the peptones and phosphates so necessary to the construction of flesh and bone in consumption and wasting diseases. It will, single-handed, sustain life. It stimulates without reaction, removing the tired, languid, exhausted feeling of delicate women, clergymen and brain workers. It dissolves and assimilates the food when taken WITH the meals, and rebuilds the worn-out mental and physical forces. It is a perfect Blood, Brain and Nerve Food.

For Feeble Digestion, Dyspepsia, Wasting or Weakness of the Lungs, Liver, Kidneys and Urinary Organs, Mental and Physical Debility, Nervousness and Want of Sleep, Female Weakness, Exhausted Mothers, Delicate Children and the aged, and every form of Debility it is marvellous.

Ask for MALT BITTERS prepared by the MALT BITTERS COMPANY, and put up in round bottles, labelled and capped as per fac-simile. Look for the MALT BITTERS COMPANY'S Signature before purchasing, and buy no other. MALT BITTERS are sold by all dealers.

MALT BITTERS COMPANY, BOSTON, MASS.

N. B.—"This is the House that Jack Built" Cards may be obtained at all gists, or mailed on receipt of three-cent stamp.

Traveling drug salesmen peddled drugs like "malt bitters," a "blood, brain, and nerve food" that offered "stimulation without intoxication." When medicines like these did not contain alcohol, they often contained cocaine instead.

was the state of affairs when the first antidepressants were developed in the 1950s.

Many pharmaceutical companies and researchers after World War II had focused on developing new antihistamines for allergy relief. By the 1950s, several effective antihistamines had already been discovered, including Benadryl® (diphenhydramine hydrochloride), which is still one of the most

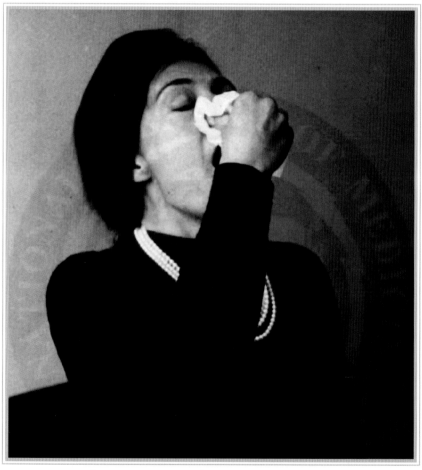

In the 1950s, researchers looking for allergy treatments developed antihistamines.

commonly used antihistamines. Despite the success of several of the early antihistamines, pharmaceutical companies continued their search for ever more effective antihistamine drugs.

One of the more common practices of the time was to examine chemicals similar in structure to drugs that had already been shown to have antihistamic effects. Through various chemical and physical transformations of these preexisting medicines, researchers were often able to discover other drugs that they would then test in a variety of ways. Often, the new compounds proved less effective than the original, but even these could be useful for the sake of research. By comparing the effects of different chemical compounds of similar natures, researchers were slowly able to put together pieces of the puzzle of how the human body works. While not every new chemical that was **synthesized** from older drugs was effective, some new drugs that proved to be more effective or had fewer side effects were generated in this way.

In the early 1950s, pharmaceutical researchers made a huge discovery that would have a tremendous impact on many different fields of medicine. That discovery was Thorazine (chlorpromazine), which would become the world's first widely used antipsychotic drug.

Thorazine was not a new drug. It had originally been used as an antihistamine and an antiemetic (a drug to prevent vomiting). Years after it had been introduced on the market, researchers working with Thorazine noticed that it seemed to have some sort of mental effects on patients with psychological disorders.

Further testing was performed on animals, which was something of an *innovation* in the field of psychiatry. While animal testing had long been an established practice in drug development, researchers generally looked only at the physical effects of a drug on the animal. In the case of Thorazine, researchers monitored the behavior of those animals—mostly rats—that were administered Thorazine. Their findings indicated that Thorazine did, in fact, have a psychological effect. Testing then proceeded in human patients, where it was found that Thorazine was very effective in combating some of the symptoms of *schizophrenia* (such as delusions, hallucinations, and paranoia).

The development of Thorazine was incredibly important for the later development of antidepressants. It marked the opening of a new field of medical research called psychopharmacology—the study of medicines used in the treatment of mental and emotional disorders such as depression. While Thorazine was the first psychiatric medicine to achieve widespread use, it was not the first such medicine to be used.

Before Thorazine, psychiatrists treating mental and emotional disorders had a few other tools at their disposal. A number of drugs had been developed prior to Thorazine that were effective in treating schizophrenia, which was the most common psychiatric diagnosis in those days. Of these, lithium and reserpine were the two most effective. For various reasons, including adverse side effects, these two drugs never achieved widespread use. More commonly used was a technique known as electroconvulsive therapy, or ECT. ECT

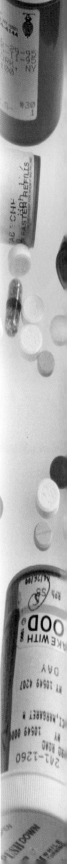

uses electrical currents to induce a brief **seizure** in the patient's brain. While this sort of treatment sounds harsh and dangerous, in reality it has been shown to be highly effective and generally safe. (ECT figures prominently—and very negatively—in Ken Kesey's *One Flew Over the Cuckoo's Nest*, where it is used to treat patients in an asylum.) Another common treatment for psychological disorders in the 1950s was psychotherapy, sometimes called "talk therapy" because the

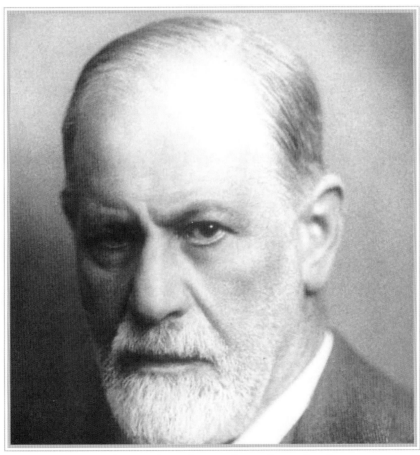

Sigmund Freud is the Father of Psychotherapy, which first became popular in the 1950s.

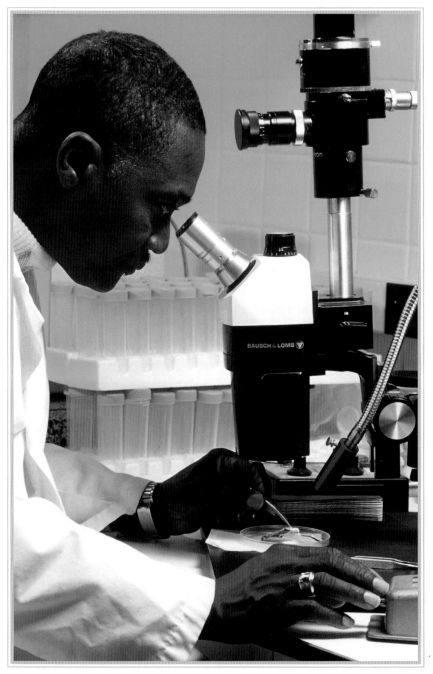

Scientific research plays an important role in both the world's health and the world's economy.

patient talks to a psychologist in order to work through issues underlying his condition.

While each of these different forms of treatment had been shown to be effective, Thorazine quickly became the treatment option of choice for many medical professionals. It required less time and effort than ECT or psychotherapy, and it appeared at the time to be more effective and safer than other drug treatments. Its success helped pave the way for the development of antidepressants.

Development of the First Antidepressants

Thorazine opened many physicians' eyes to the possibility that medicines could be used to treat psychological disorders. Still, most people didn't believe that medications could treat something such as depression, which most experts believed was a reaction to a social stimulus, such as loss. Perhaps that's why it took so long for the first antidepressants to be discovered. Like Thorazine, these drugs were actually first developed to treat other conditions.

In 1957, two very different drugs were approved in Europe for the treatment of depression. One of these two drugs, Tofranil, owed a great deal to Thorazine. Like Thorazine, Tofranil had initially been developed as an antihistamine. In fact, both Tofranil and Thorazine had been synthesized from the same basic chemical, phenothiazine, which has since become the basis for many different antihistamines and antipsychotic drugs. For this reason, the two drugs have a nearly identical three-ring chemical structure.

Once the use of Thorazine as an antipsychotic became established, researchers working on Tofranil began to wonder if the similar chemical structure of Tofranil would equate to similar therapeutic effects. Testing of Tofranil on human subjects began in the mid-1950s and were originally inconclusive. Many of the researchers, after all, did not believe a drug could have an antidepressant effect, and so they weren't looking for one. In fact, in healthy patients, Tofranil has a slightly sedative effect, quite the opposite of what one might expect from an antidepressant. Nevertheless, researchers eventually did discover the antidepressant effects of Tofranil, and the drug was soon marketed as an antidepressant.

The other antidepressant drug that was released in 1957 was Marsilid. Marsilid did not share the same commonalities with Thorazine that Tofranil did. Whereas the latter two drugs had been originally developed as antihistamines and were derived from phenothiazine, Marsilid began its life as a treatment for *tuberculosis*. What's more, Marsilid was derived from rocket fuel.

After World War II, chemical and pharmaceutical companies began experimenting with surplus German rocket fuel called hydrazine. Performing chemical transformations on hydrazine produced a variety of different chemical compounds, including Marsilid, which researchers discovered had some effect on managing tuberculosis. Testing of Marsilid seemed to show that it was promising, and it was eventually approved for use against tuberculosis.

Doctors using Marsilid on their patients, however, noticed that the drug appeared to have some psychological side effects. Patients taking Marsilid seemed to have more energy and seemed to gain some weight when taking the drug, both of which were very desirable effects. At the time, the antipsychotic effects of Thorazine had not yet been discovered, and doctors and researchers did not consider that Marsilid could

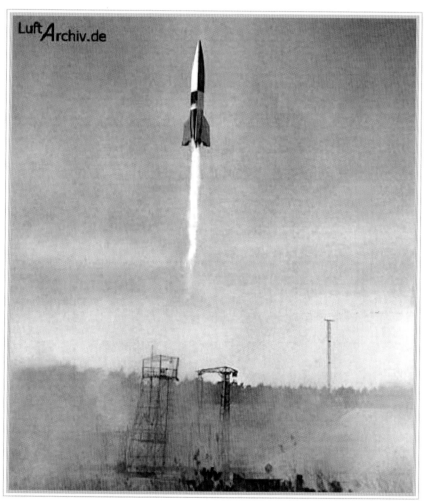

Surprisingly, the development of German rocket fuel during World War II eventually led to one of the first antidepressants.

have an antidepressant effect. They did notice that people using the drug tended to have more energy, but they believed this was a result of the weight gain. For this reason, testing then began on Marsilid as a nutritional aid to help patients gain weight. It was not until after it became clear that Thorazine was an effective antipsychotic that researchers finally realized the antidepressant effect of Marsilid. Although the drug had already been on the market for several years for the treatment of tuberculosis, Marsilid did not gain approval as an antidepressant until about the same time as Tofranil did.

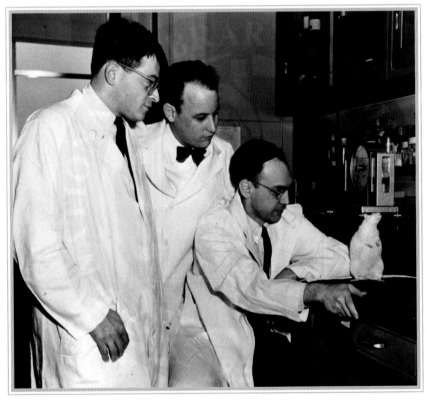

Research done on rats has its limitations, since obviously, the rat can't report on its emotional state.

The examples of how Tofranil and Marsilid were developed show how drugs were traditionally discovered and brought to market. As with most drugs of that time, testing of the early antidepressants began on animals, mostly lab rats. These rats were observed for behavioral changes and for any physical effects the drugs might have caused. These tests gave the researchers some basic idea of the effects of the drugs, though this understanding was by no means complete. After all, while researchers could observe certain behaviors and measurable physical effects in the rats, they could not very well expect answers to simple questions about how the rats felt while taking the medicines! For these answers, the researchers had to turn to human subjects.

Prior to the Kefauver-Harris Amendment of 1962, drug testing had the potential of being quite a dangerous process. Researchers administered varying doses of their experimental drug to human subjects, who they then monitored just as they had monitored the rats. People who volunteered for these tests, however, ran a rather serious risk. While researchers could calculate rough estimates on the amount of the drug required for a lethal dose, these estimates ignored a great many variables. Testing for lethality in rats could give researchers only a rough idea of the safe limits of a drug. Furthermore, some of the side effects of an experimental drug could not yet have been determined properly. Nor, for that matter, was the proper therapeutic dose established at the time of human testing. A human test subject could be receiving far more of the medication than was necessary in order to achieve effective therapeutic results, which could result in more adverse side effects.

The examples of Tofranil and Marsilid are also helpful in better understanding how the drugs are discovered in the first place. In the 1950s, the technology did not exist that would allow drug developers to accurately predict the effects of a given chemical compound on the human body. Drug development, therefore, was a matter of trial and error. A chemical compound would be tested on lab rats, and its effects would be observed. If those effects seemed useful or promising, then researchers would further pursue that compound. Otherwise, they would record their data and move on to another compound. Discovering new drugs at that time was more a matter of luck and patience than it was of skill.

While luck and patience are still important factors in the drug discovery process, recent advances in technology and science have made it far easier for drug developers to focus their efforts on chemical compounds that are more likely to yield positive results.

Advances in Drug Development

Tofranil and Marsilid opened the way for other antidepressant drugs to follow. Throughout the 1960s and 1970s, tricyclic antidepressants—such as Tofranil and Elavil® (amitriptyline hydrochloride)—and MAOI antidepressants—such as Marsilid and Nardil® (phenelzine sulfate)—had decent success as medical options for the treatment of depression. These early antidepressants, however, had a variety of adverse side effects, making some doctors hesitant to prescribe them.

In 1987, Prozac was introduced in the United States, ushering in a revolution in the treatment of depression that was, in many ways, just as important as the original development of the first antidepressants. Unlike the earlier generations of antidepressants, Prozac had very few serious negative side effects. Doctors felt comfortable in prescribing it in a variety of situations. Whereas the older antidepressants were generally reserved only for the most serious cases of depression, Prozac and the newer SSRIs that followed it could be used even for patients suffering from mild depression.

The way in which Prozac was developed also marked a significant change in the process by which antidepressants and other drugs are developed. To a certain extent, this change

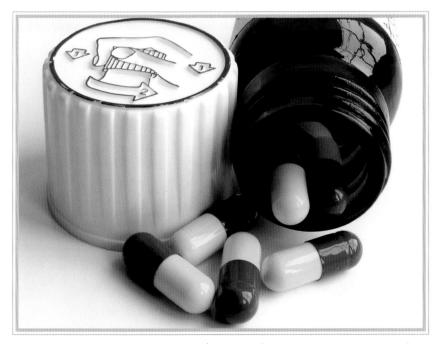

Prozac revolutionized the way depression was treated.

occurred as a result of new guidelines established in the 1962 Kefauver-Harris Amendment to the Food, Drug, and Cosmetics Act regarding drug development and testing. More important, however, developments in pharmaceutical technology and science gave drug developers powerful new tools that changed the way they formulated new drugs.

Prozac was the first original antidepressant to be designed specifically for the treatment of depression. Recall that the early tricyclics and MAOIs had been designed for purposes other than the treatment of depression. Later generations of

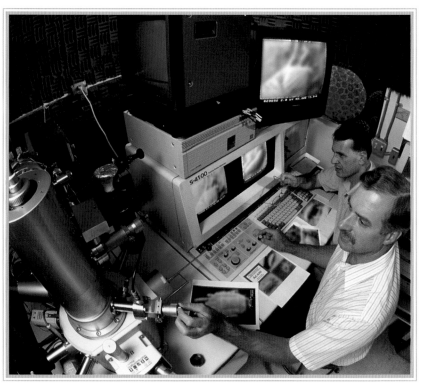

Technological advances have allowed researchers to better understand some of the factors that influence drug development.

these types of antidepressants were designed for the treatment of depression, but they were essentially just **derivatives** of their predecessors. Prozac, on the other hand, had been planned out from the beginning as an antidepressant, even before anybody could test it to see its effects.

This was possible because advances in technology and science allowed scientists to better understand several key factors in the development of a drug. The first of these is body mechanics—the ways in which the human body regulates itself and the processes by which it functions. Earlier generations of antidepressants had made it clear to researchers that several chemicals, called amines, are important in determining mood, motivation, and energy. Scientists singled out one of these amines—serotonin—as a key chemical in warding off depression. Thus, when drug developers set out to create Prozac, they knew they wanted to produce a drug that could boost serotonin levels in the brain.

Another tool available to modern drug developers is an improved understanding of chemistry, as well as the computing power necessary to model complex chemical compounds. Knowing that the brain needed more serotonin to overcome depression was only useful if developers could find some chemical that addressed that need. When researchers first began designing Prozac, the computing power they could bring to bear on the problem paled in comparison to today's standards. Still, the combined advances in chemistry and computing gave developers unprecedented insight into the nature and effects of Prozac's chemical formulation.

Of course, projections and predictions can only tell scientists so much about a chemical, its effectiveness, and the safety of using it. Testing is still a critical component of the overall drug development process. By testing a drug like Prozac on laboratory rats, developers are able to get a better idea of how the drug works, what side effects it causes, and what sort of adverse reactions it creates when taken in conjunction with other drugs. For some, the thought of using animals such as rats in drug experiments seems **inhumane**. On the other hand, some of the drugs that are tested will go on to become lifesaving or life-enhancing drugs.

Drug Development Today

Today, the drug development process relies very heavily on computers running simulations, projections, and models. This has helped make the process much more streamlined and efficient, but it has also helped make it much more expensive.

Financial analysts estimate that the current cost of developing a new drug lies somewhere in the range of 500 million to 800 million dollars. That's ten times more than the entire pharmaceutical industry in North America made in revenues a century ago. In 2002 alone, pharmaceutical companies in the United States spent an estimated 31 billion dollars on research and development. Some of that money was spent testing existing drugs, but a significant portion was spent on bringing new drugs to market.

Drug development is not only a costly process, but it is also a very time-consuming one. On average, a new drug spends its first three to four years in what are called preclinical trials. These trials show the developing pharmaceutical company whether a chemical compound appears to be promising. In the case of antidepressants, for example, preclinical trials might give developers an idea of whether a new drug raises levels of certain amines in the brain. The preclinical trials also help to give developers some dosing guidelines, and help them establish safe dosing limits. At this point in a drug's development, the drug is not tested on human subjects.

Generally, at some point during preclinical trials, the pharmaceutical company developing the new drug will apply for a patent. This protects the company from having their drug copied by a competitor, which gives them some security on the heavy investment they are making in developing the drug.

When developers are satisfied that their chemical compound will make an effective drug, they apply to the FDA to begin testing the drug clinically. This application is called an investigational new drug application, or IND for short. If the IND is accepted, then the drug can begin clinical testing, putting it one step closer to becoming a marketed drug. Clinical testing, however, is an extremely long process.

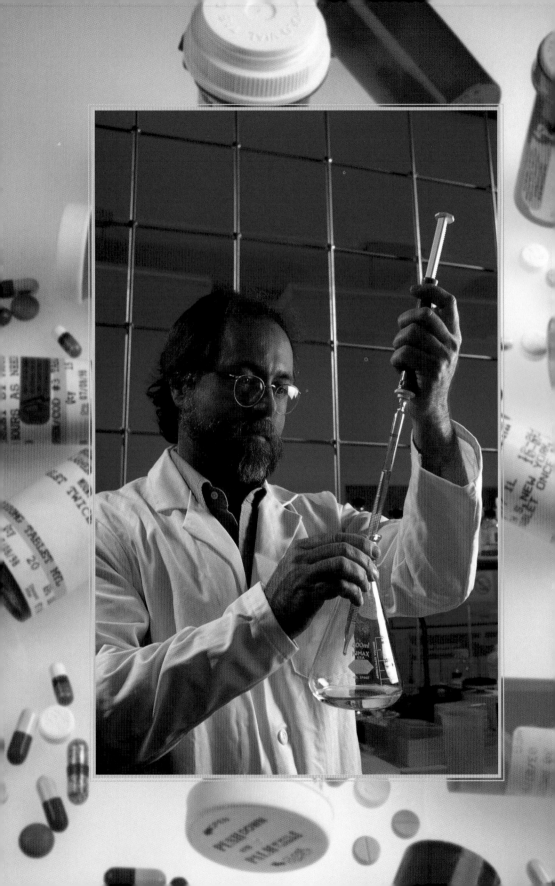

Chapter 4

The Drug Approval Process

*D*rug development alone is a costly, lengthy, and often frustrating process. It is only half the story behind bringing a new drug to market, however. The other half of that story is the drug approval process, which in many ways guides the drug development process.

Before a company can begin selling a medicine, that medicine must first be approved by the FDA for use as a treatment for a given condition. Prozac, for instance, had to be approved for use in the treatment of depression before it could be sold as an antidepressant. The process of securing that approval begins in preclinical trials. The three to four years a drug might spend in preclinical trials, however, is only a small part of the overall drug approval process.

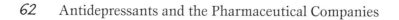

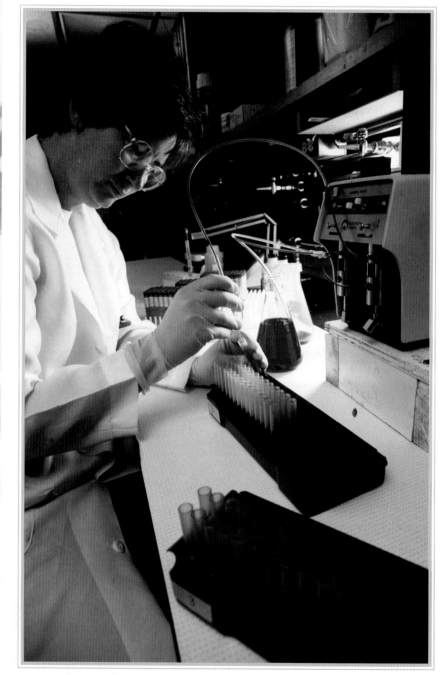

Clinical trials use samples from human beings to determine appropriate doses for a medication.

Once an investigational new drug receives approval, the company developing it can move on to clinical trials. These trials are broken up into three phases.

Clinical Trial Phase 1

The first phase of a clinical trial focuses primarily on establishing proper dosing guidelines and determining whether a drug is safe to use. Some preliminary information in this regard would have been gleaned from preclinical trials. That information, however, would have come from tests of the drug on animals, and so it might not be accurate for humans.

In order to determine the proper dosing and safety guidelines in humans, human volunteers are employed in the first clinical trial phase. In general, somewhere between twenty to a hundred volunteers are chosen to receive the experimental drug. These volunteers are generally healthy rather than people suffering from the condition the drug is intended to treat. In cases where the drug is intended to treat a life-threatening sickness such as AIDS, the FDA will allow the testing company to employ volunteers with the condition only if no other proven treatment is available. While a condition like depression is serious, other treatments are available. Thus, volunteers in phase one clinical trials for antidepressants are healthy people who do not have depression.

At this point in the trial, the doses given to the trial subjects are kept low for the sake of safety. Over the course of the trial, the doses are slowly increased. This method allows researchers to monitor the test subjects closely for any signs of adverse reactions and for signs that the medicine is working. This helps to prevent dangerous reactions to the medicine and allows developers more control over any **variables** that might affect the drug's safety and effectiveness.

Phase one clinical trials generally take about one year to complete, though they may take longer. Approximately 70 percent of investigational new drugs will continue on to phase two. The pharmaceutical company generally discontinues 30 percent for any of a variety of reasons. The medicine may prove to be too dangerous to use in humans, or its negative side effects outweigh the positive benefits of using the drug. At any rate, by weeding out obviously ineffective and dangerous drugs, the first clinical trial phase helps to ensure that drugs brought to market are both safe and effective for use.

Clinical Trial Phase 2

The second phase of clinical testing focuses on determining whether the investigational drug is effective. In this phase, one hundred to three hundred volunteers are recruited to take the experimental medication. Because the goal is to determine whether the medicine is effective, these volunteers are all people with the condition the drug is intended to treat. In the case of antidepressants, then, phase two trial subjects are all people with depression.

As in the first phase, subjects start off taking very low doses of the drug, and then slowly work their way up to higher doses. Researchers use this opportunity to monitor a number of different variables. One factor researchers examine at this

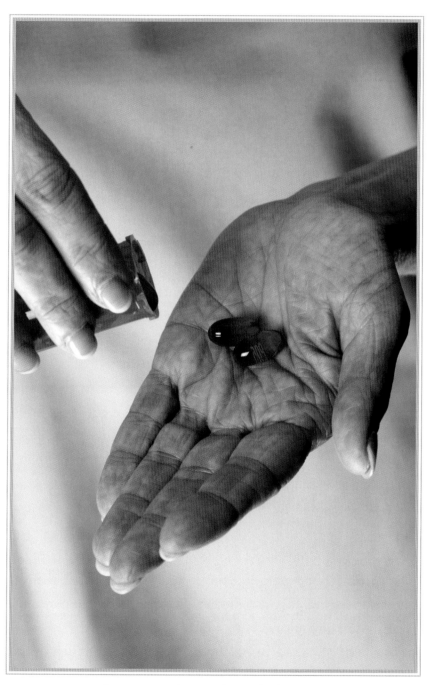

Phase-two clinical trials determine whether the medication is effective.

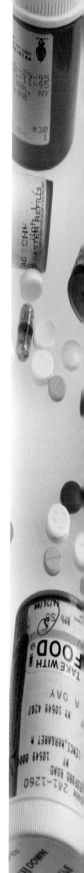

point is the method of drug delivery—that is, whether the drug is best taken in pill form, as a liquid, as an injection, or as an inhaler. Researchers can then get a better idea of which method of delivery works the fastest, which is most effective, which lasts longest, and so on.

Another important consideration at this point is determining the dosing interval, which indicates how often the medicine should be taken for maximum effectiveness. This can be determined in a number of ways, including monitoring the concentrations of the drug in subjects' blood, as well as simply by observing its effects in subjects using the drug at different dosing intervals. An important aspect of determining the dosing interval is once again verifying the safety of the experimental drug.

Phase two testing occurs over the course of, on average, one to two years. Despite the time put into testing the drugs that make it to this point in the development process, many of them will not pass on to the third phase. Of the 70 percent of investigational new drugs that pass the first clinical phase, about half will not pass the second phase. Only 33 percent of INDs will make it to clinical trial phase three.

Clinical Trial Phase 3

The third clinical phase is the longest of the three clinical phases of testing. It is also the last phase before an experimental drug can be approved for sale.

In the third phase, researchers work to verify much of the information accumulated in the first two phases of clinical testing. Once again, researchers work to verify the safety and efficacy of the test drug. In addition, using data collected from phase two, they attempt to determine the best dosage for the drug. This is made possible by the length of the third phase trials, which can be anywhere from three to ten years.

During that time, researchers work with a much larger pool of test volunteers—generally between one thousand to three thousand people in many different locations across the country. In the first two clinical trial phases, the volunteers are people who come in to a test center to participate in the

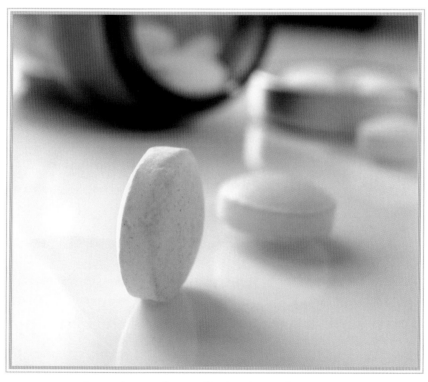

During phase-three clinical trials, as many as three thousand volunteers take the medication to help researchers determine the best dosage.

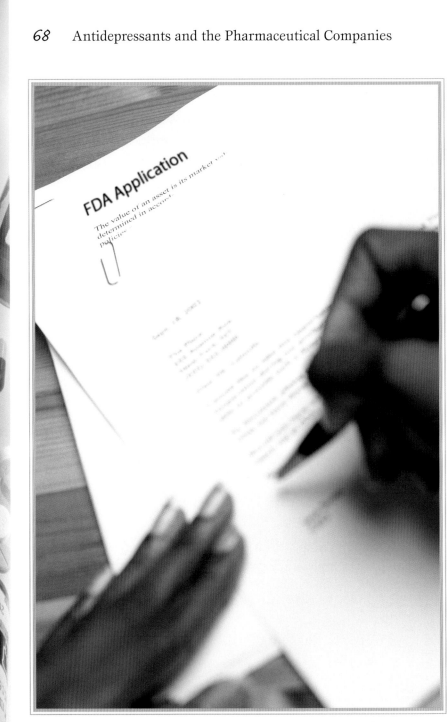

Once the clinical testing is completed, the pharmaceutical company must submit detailed paper records of all test results to the FDA.

study, and the people administering the drug are usually professional researchers. Any variable in the first two phases is tightly controlled so the researchers can study specific aspects of the test drug. In the third phase, however, practicing doctors administer the drug to standard patients, be it in a hospital or in the doctor's general practice.

The benefit of this approach to third phase testing is that it allows for a greater variety of variables in the study, which makes a greater range of responses to the drug possible. This allows researchers to get a much better idea of how the drug interacts with other substances in the human body, how it affects the body over the long term, and whom the drug will benefit most.

At the end of clinical testing, the pharmaceutical company that is developing the new drug gathers all of the data it has collected thus far on the experimental drug, fills out a great deal of paperwork, and submits an application to the FDA for drug approval. This application is called, appropriately enough, a new drug application—NDA. The NDA includes not only all of the information—both negative and positive— about the drug, but also the company's proposed package labeling.

Despite all the work that a company puts into the development of the drug to this point, the FDA will not approve about 10 percent of INDs that make it to phase three trials. Many other NDAs will be denied because paperwork is filed incorrectly or the company has neglected to submit certain important information. Applications that are denied for this reason can be resubmitted with the appropriate corrections, but the delay proves expensive for the company. Any time that the drug is not being sold is time that the company is losing money on that drug.

The FDA must review a tremendous amount of information in the NDA—as much as seventeen years' worth of data collected in clinical and preclinical trials. For that reason, it often takes the FDA a long time to review a new application.

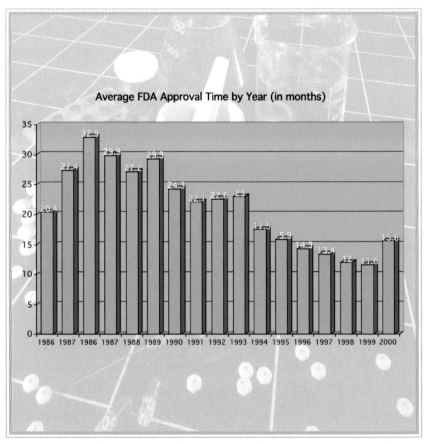

The FDA has reduced its approval time significantly since 1986, but the process still takes a year or more.

In 2000, the FDA spent an average of 15.6 months reviewing each NDA. At the end of that time, the FDA makes a decision as to whether the drug will be approved. If it is approved, the company that produced the drug can begin selling it. If not, the company must decide what to do with the drug. Many drugs that fail to earn approval will become valuable research aids for future drug development. Due to the expense of drug development, however, a drug that fails in the third clinical phase results in a tremendous financial loss for the company that produced it. Drug development, while important and potentially lucrative, is by no means without its risks.

Post-Marketing Trials

Although a drug has already been approved for sale, the scrutiny focused on it does not end there. The clinical trial process is a very comprehensive method of data collection. However, it is by no means perfect. A drug that appears safe and effective in a controlled study of a few thousand volunteers might prove dangerous when used on a larger scale, where chances are more side effects may appear. Once on the market, the drug may also be used in combination with certain foods or drugs that none of the volunteers in the studies used. In addition, certain problems regarding drugs only become apparent after a person has been using it for many years. The relatively short time frame imposed by the clinical trial process makes it difficult to provide this sort of long-term study.

For that reason, drugs continue to be studied even after they have been released on the market. These studies take

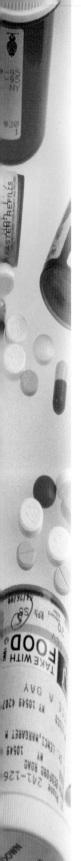

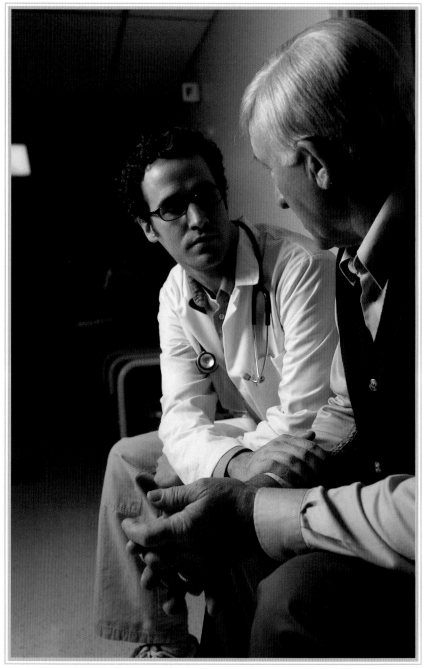

As doctors observe patients' reactions to new drugs, they report any serious side effects to the FDA.

two forms. First, the pharmaceutical company that produced the drug could call for another clinical study. This is often referred to as a "phase four" trial, since it follows very much in the footsteps of the pre-approval clinical trials. Studies of this sort often focus on more specific conditions than the clinical trials required in the drug approval process. In the case of antidepressants, the FDA might ask a pharmaceutical company to test its product in a specific population or age group, or even in a group that has another medical condition—say, high blood pressure, for example. These studies are used to better understand how best to use the drug and to verify its safety once again.

Another, more common type of surveillance that all drugs must undergo is public perception. Doctors who prescribe a

Is the FDA Doing Its Job?

Recently, the FDA has been under criticism for not monitoring medications carefully enough after they're on the market. For example, the FDA allowed the anti-inflammatory drugs Vioxx® and Bextra® to stay on the market for years, despite reports that they caused an increased risk of heart problems or stroke. In 2004, however, the FDA asked Pfizer to stop selling Bextra, and in 2004 Merck agreed to withdraw Vioxx from pharmacy shelves. The FDA has vowed to increase its ongoing scrutiny of approved medications.

medicine and notice any serious adverse side effects or reactions are required to report those reactions to the FDA program called Medwatch. Every three months after a drug is approved, the manufacturer must report any known instances of side effects to the FDA. All this information is then used to further analyze the effectiveness and safety of the drug, as well as to promote safe use of that drug.

As reports about side effects and adverse reactions become available, drug labeling is amended to include this information. In extreme cases, the FDA can require pharmaceutical companies to post warnings about a drug on that drug's label. This happened in the case of several of the SSRIs. In 2004, the FDA required manufacturers of all SSRIs to include a "black box" warning regarding an increased risk of suicide among people taking them for depression. The black box warning is an indication of very serious and potentially dangerous side effects from the use of a particular drug. It was added to SSRIs due to an increase in the incidence of suicide attempts among people—particularly young people—using antidepressants.

Clearly, the FDA's decision to order black box warnings about suicide on SSRI package labeling did not please the manufacturers of those medicines. Perhaps, however, they should have felt fortunate. The FDA is also charged with the power to withdraw a medicine from the market if that drug poses a substantial health threat to people using it. In 1986, just one year after it was released on the markets, the antidepressant Wellbutrin® (bupropion hydrochloride) was recalled after doctors discovered that many patients had seizures after

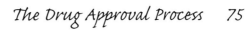

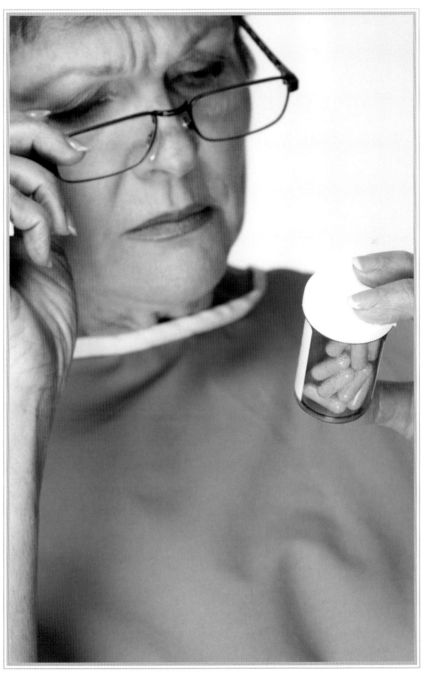

Drug companies must obey the FDA's regulations regarding how their drugs are labeled.

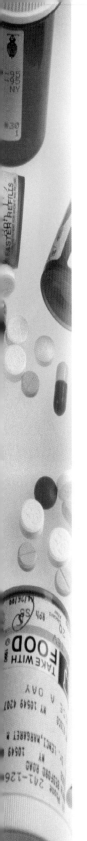

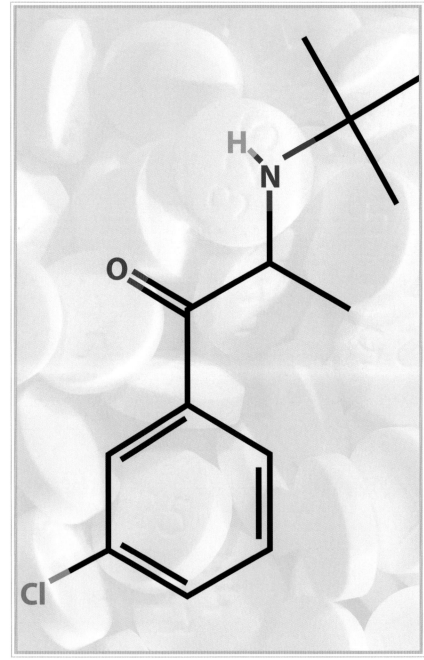

Although Wellbutrin is still used to treat depression, Prozac is better known.

using the medicine. Further clinical tests after its withdrawal showed that a lower dose of Wellbutrin reduced the risk of seizures without compromising its effectiveness in combating depression. The drug was re-released on the market in 1989 for use as an antidepressant. It was also approved in 1997 as an aid in quitting smoking. Although it has the same chemical formulation, this form of the drug is better known as Zyban®.

Wellbutrin might have been known as the drug that revolutionized the treatment of depression if not for its withdrawal from the market. One year after Wellbutrin was withdrawn, Prozac entered the market. It was Prozac—not Wellbutrin—that became an *icon* of American culture. It was Prozac—not Wellbutrin—that revolutionized the treatment of depression. And while most people who were treated for depression at that time probably weren't too concerned with which medicine they used so long as it worked, the companies and their stockholders that watched this drama unfold witnessed a pivotal moment in the modern pharmaceutical industry.

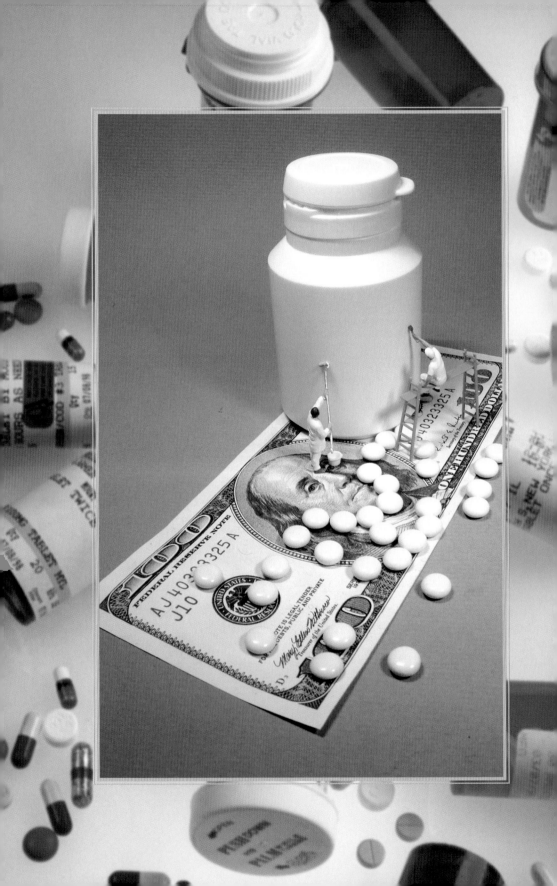

Chapter 5

The Bottom Line: Corporate Responsibilities to Shareholders

*T*o this point, we have considered the medicines produced by the pharmaceutical companies as an end in themselves. That is to say, we have looked at medicine as the purpose of the pharmaceutical industry, the goal toward which the industry works. Such an analysis, however, is not entirely accurate.

While it is true that the pharmaceutical industry has done a great deal of good in the world by creating medicines to combat disease and sickness, to alleviate pain, and to help people with psychological disorders like depression regain normality in their lives, the industry is not merely a vehicle for creating cures. It is a business as well. As such, one of the primary motivations of the pharmaceutical industry must be profit.

Financial Outlooks

Over the past decade, the pharmaceutical industry has experienced remarkable business growth. From 1999 to 2000 alone, revenues from the sales of prescription drugs increased about 19 percent, from 111.1 billion dollars in 1999 to 132 billion dollars in 2000. From 1997 to 2005, the industry enjoyed an annual rate of growth of more than 10 percent.

Part of this is due to the increasingly effective drugs the industry is creating. Conditions once considered difficult or impossible to treat can now be controlled through advanced ***drug regimens***. Even conditions that were not considered medical conditions in the past can now be remedied through the use of medicines. Depression, obesity, and high cholesterol are all examples of conditions that were once considered lifestyle issues but that are now thought of as serious but treatable medical problems.

To some extent, problems such as these have become recognized medically because of the efforts of the pharmaceutical industry. The case of antidepressants, in particular, illustrates how the industry has created a market for a product. Prior to the introduction of antidepressants, physicians and psychiatrists rarely diagnosed depression. To some extent, this reflects advances in the field of psychology. Pharmaceutical promotions, however, have done a great deal to promote an awareness of depression among general physicians, who are, not coincidentally, the people responsible for diagnosing depression and prescribing antidepressants.

After the introduction of Prozac and several other SSRIs such as Zoloft and Paxil, the market for antidepressants began to shoot upward. Between 2000 and 2001, antidepressant sales grew at a faster rate than any other class of medicine. The last major update to the guidelines for diagnosing depression came in 1994, in the *Diagnostic and Statistical Manual of Mental Disorders, Fourth Edition*, known more commonly as the DSM-IV. This manual serves as the basis by which all psychological disorders, including depression, are diagnosed. While the DSM-IV was available in 1994, not until several years later did the number of prescriptions for antidepressants really began to skyrocket.

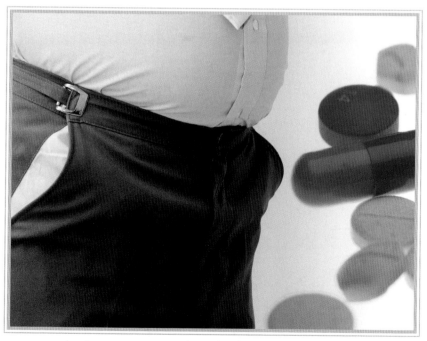

Obesity, once considered a lifestyle issue, is now treated with medication, just as depression is.

In 1997, remember, the FDA loosened the restrictions against DTC advertising of prescription medications, bringing information about depression and antidepressants to general consumers for the first time through mass media. In 1996, before the FDA permitted DTC advertising of prescription drugs, the pharmaceutical industry spent about 800 million dollars on DTC advertising. This figure represented the limited amount of advertising that was permissible under the law. By 2000, after those restrictions were eased, that number had risen to approximately 2.5 billion dollars, a threefold increase over five years. Revenues throughout the industry began to increase rapidly as a result.

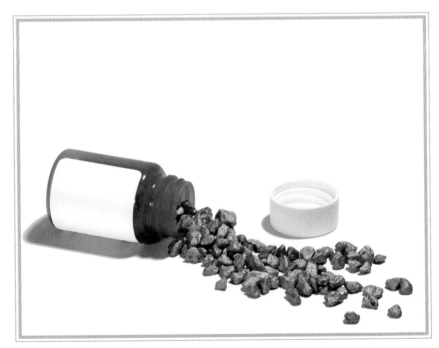

Antidepressants are the pharmaceutical companies' "gold mine."

Antidepressants became one of the more heavily advertised classes of drugs, and one of the more lucrative. Today, you can see advertisements on television, in magazines, and on the Internet promoting various brands of antidepressants. Such exposure has vaulted antidepressant brands like Prozac, Zoloft, and Paxil into stratospheric sales. In 1999 alone, those three drugs accounted for nearly 7 billion dollars worth of sales. With sales figures like that, it's little wonder that *Fortune* magazine listed the pharmaceutical industry as the most profitable industry in the United States in 2001.

Such success, however, has riled many critics. They contend that the pharmaceutical industry is profiting from the suffering of other people, and that the industry unfairly and unethically inflates the prices of drugs in order to enhance its own profits. These people believe that the high-revenue growth of the pharmaceutical industry over the past decade has been a result of patented medicines that are priced too expensively, the costs of DTC advertising, and the influence of the pharmaceutical industry over the prescribing habits of doctors. Older (and cheaper drugs) may be equally effective— but pharmaceutical companies advertise the newer, costlier drugs. As a result, doctors and hospitals may not prescribe the older, cheaper, but equally effective medications.

Justifications for High Revenues

Like any industry, the pharmaceutical industry relies on profits to grow and expand. Whereas companies in some other industries expand by opening new stores or sales outlets, pharmaceutical companies expand by developing a wider variety of medicines. This expansion, they maintain, is essential to the continued advancement of health care.

Does this, however, answer the criticism that pharmaceutical companies intentionally set their prices too high? The high cost of prescription drugs is a major drain on the economy of North America, and in particular the United States. In 2002, American expenditures on drugs totaled about 200 billion dollars. That marked an increase of more than 8 percent over spending on drugs in the previous year. Spending on health insurance rose even faster, by 10 percent over the previous year (faster than the rate of inflation). Taken together, we see that total health-care expenditures are becoming an increasingly heavy burden on North American consumers.

On the other hand, it's important to remember that new drugs remain patent protected for only a limited time. During the patent life of a brand name drug, a company can expect to make significant profits on their product, because at that time the company that produced the product enjoys exclusive sales rights. After the patent life on a drug expires, however, less expensive generic copies quickly devour the market for that drug. Although the patent life of a drug is twenty years and can be extended under certain circumstances, by the time most drugs gain approval from the FDA, they have only about ten to twelve years of patent life remaining. Thus, drug companies need to be able to make their money back quickly.

In the case of Prozac, Eli Lilly—the company that makes Prozac—made a whopping 21 billion dollars from sales of the

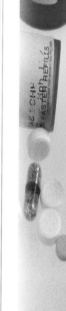

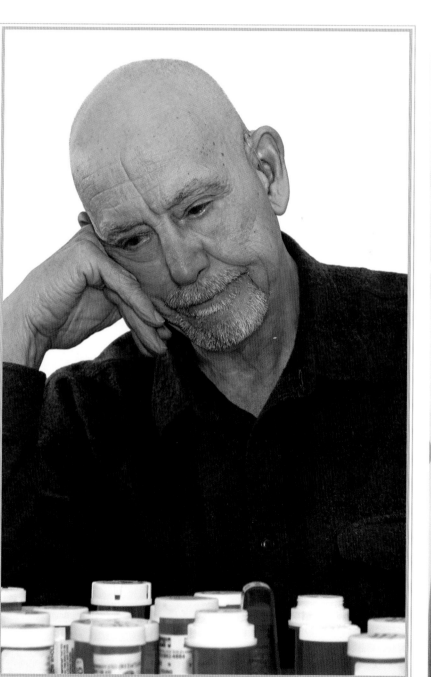

*Ultimately, consumers are the ones who pay
pharmaceutical companies' profits.*

medicine during its patent life. Prozac is one of the best-selling drugs in the history of the pharmaceutical industry. Within a month of losing patent protection, though, fully 80 percent of Prozac's sales had been lost to generic competitors. Sales of Prozac dropped from roughly 200 million dollars per month to about four million dollars per month.

Clearly, however, Prozac had more than recouped its development cost by the time it reached that point. In fact, it

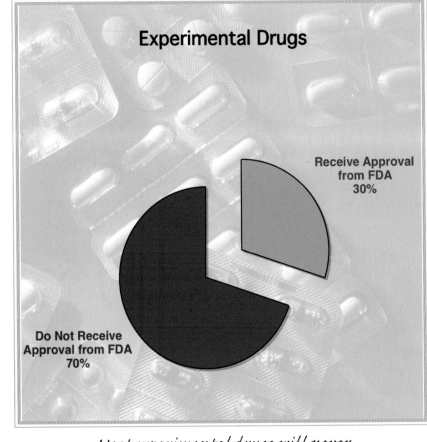

Most experimental drugs will never receive approval from the FDA.

paid for its development cost several times over. During the time that Prozac was being sold, however, Eli Lilly was not simply counting its profits. The pharmaceutical company was busy developing other drugs, both antidepressants and other classes of drugs. The money coming from the sale of Prozac was paying for the development of new drugs. Keep in mind too that fully 70 percent of experimental drugs never gain approval from the FDA to be marketed. Many—in fact, most—of the drugs that pharmaceutical companies begin to develop will not be profitable. Many will never even be sold. For this reason, pharmaceutical industry advocates maintain, the high cost of drugs is reasonable. Without profits, new drug development would halt.

What's more, drugs that are developed in the United States generate enormous profits at home—but they are sold around the world for much less than they are in American pharmacies. This means the people in third-world nations in Africa, Asia, and South America benefit because these drugs were developed. In a way, American consumers fund the entire world's drug research.

The Role of the Shareholder

Profits fuel not only new drug development, however. Profits, in general, fuel business growth and the confidence that stockbrokers place in a company. For good or bad, the corporate environment of today places a great deal of emphasis on a company's bottom line—the company's ability to make money.

Because many pharmaceutical companies are publicly traded companies—meaning anybody can buy shares of their stock, in essence becoming part owners in the companies—company executives are charged with the responsibility of ensuring the growth of revenues and profits. Failure to do so causes the price of a stock to fall, which causes shareholders to lose money. Since shareholders typically don't enjoy losing money, that puts pressure on the companies to perform well financially. Some critics argue that this pressure causes the industry to increase drug prices even beyond what is necessary to develop new drugs.

Whatever the case, there are no easy answers on the issue. Understandably, debate continues over whether the pharmaceutical industry is focusing too much on their bottom line and not enough on providing inexpensive treatment options for patients. So long as there is money to be made in pharmaceuticals and people who want to feel better, the debate will probably continue.

University Research

Not all drugs are developed solely by big corporations; research also take place at academic centers. In some cases, federal, state, university, and industry funds all contribute to the creation of a medication.

Now we turn our attention toward some of the ethical controversies that have beset the industry over the past decade. Truly, in most regards, we cannot easily separate ethical issues from financial ones, since so many of these issues eventually come down to a conflict between financial gain and moral responsibility.

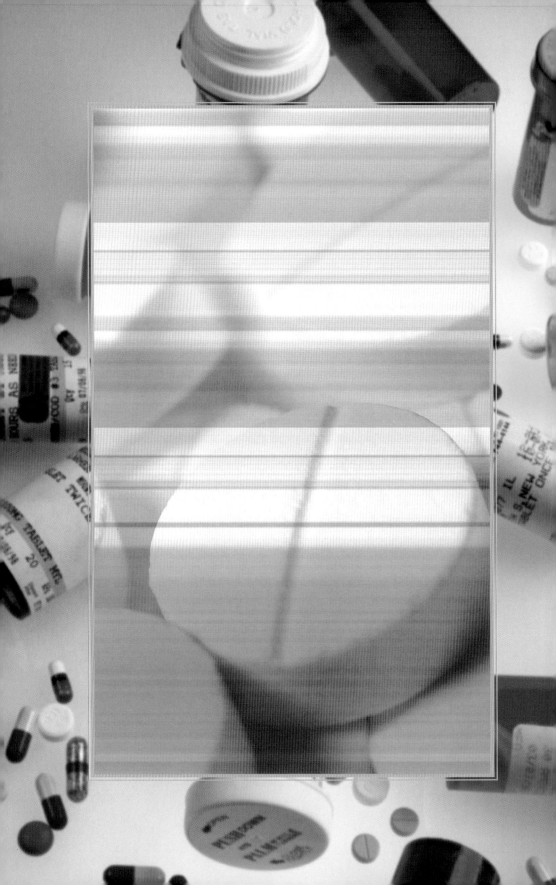

Chapter 6

Shades of Gray: Corporate Ethical Responsibilities

*I*t is easy to look back at the early pharmaceutical industry and romanticize it, thinking that perhaps the innovators of certain landmark drugs had the good of all people in mind when they discovered the drugs. In some cases, this may be what happened. It could just as well be the case today, however. After all, it is individuals and teams of scientists who discover medicines, not the corporations who hire them. While it is easy to think that the high profits and tremendous revenue growth of the pharmaceutical industry in this day and age indicate that industry leaders are more interested in profits than they once were, the pharmaceutical companies have always been businesses guided by profit.

Information Control

As we saw when we looked at the drug development and approval process, creating new drugs is an extremely information intensive endeavor. Observations regarding drug safety, dosing, efficacy, and side effects from thousands of patients are compiled to better understand how well the drug works. Molecular models, chemical interaction studies, and toxicity projections help developers predict what the drug will do and how much will be fatal. Surveys of test subjects pinpoint possible problem areas in the use of the drug and highlight potential benefits.

The company creating the drug as part of the new drug application process brings all this information together. The FDA then reviews the information provided and makes a decision as to whether the drug will be approved for use. What's more, information gathered from post-marketing trials and from the observations of practicing physicians adds to the wealth of information about a drug even after it is approved. But who is responsible for making this information public? The pharmaceutical companies are.

A recent lawsuit brings this issue to light. GlaxoSmith-Kline—the company that produces the SSRI Paxil—was sued in 2004 for withholding information that showed a possible increase in suicidal behavior among children and teenagers taking Paxil. In the face of this lawsuit, GlaxoSmithKline settled out of court. As a result of this settlement, the company was forced to disclose all of the information it had gathered regarding the safety and efficacy of Paxil—both positive and

The courts have been asked to step in and settle
whether or not pharmaceutical companies have
fulfilled their responsibilities to consumers.

negative—to the FDA. This disclosure made GlaxoSmithKline the first pharmaceutical company to divulge all this information. As public pressure increased, others followed suit.

Such lack of disclosure may unfortunately be unsettlingly common in the pharmaceutical industry. For one thing, the

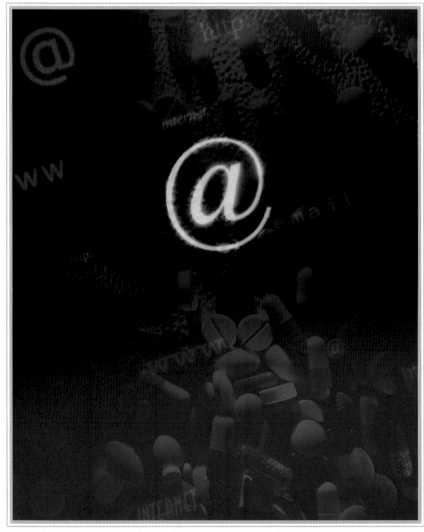

The Internet allows both doctors and consumers access to a wide range of information about medications.

massive volume of information produced by clinical trials and post-market studies would be difficult to disclose meaningfully. On the other hand, many people believe pharmaceutical companies use their influence to prevent publication of information that would be harmful to them or would hurt sales of their medicines. Pharmaceutical companies sponsor many medical and psychiatric journals by advertising in them. Journal editors, nervous about losing the financial support of the companies advertising in their journals, may be hesitant to allow the publication of any articles critical of the companies or their products. By this means, information provided to doctors and psychiatrists may be skewed in favor of the companies supporting the journals.

In addition, and perhaps more important, the companies that produce the drugs are the ones who conduct post-marketing studies. For this reason, the companies have a great deal of control over the information regarding their drugs that gets published in professional journals, which are among the top sources of medical information for doctors, psychiatrists, and pharmacists. While pharmaceutical companies are quick to publish reports and articles friendly to their products, they are equally quick to dismiss reports that portray their medicines in a negative light.

With the growth of the Internet, more information is being made available to physicians, as well as to general consumers. This information, however, can sometimes be difficult to find. Compared to the information presented in articles and advertisements—both DTC and in professional journals—the amount of information that has no industry bias appears to be fairly small. What's more, readers need to be wary of a bias in the opposite direction, by people who are critical of the pharmaceutical industry and don't present a fair picture of its position and intentions.

Some people believe the FDA should do more to regulate not only the drugs produced by the pharmaceutical industry, but also the information published. This is an unlikely solution, however, as the FDA is already extremely taxed by its responsibilities as a consumer protection agency. Currently, fully one-quarter of every dollar spent by consumers in the United States is spent on a product regulated by the FDA, be it medicine, shampoo, or food. As things are, the FDA simply doesn't have the resources to police the pharmaceutical industry more closely. Critics, however, call on the federal government to provide the FDA with the funding it needs to do a better job.

Truth in Advertising

Similar to the issue of corporate control of information regarding drug safety and efficacy is the issue of truth in advertising. The United States and New Zealand are the only two economically advanced countries in the world that currently allow DTC advertising of prescription medications, and the government of New Zealand is considering legislation to prohibit it. With the flood of advertising that resulted from the FDA's 1997 decision to loosen restrictions on DTC advertising of prescription drugs, an important consideration must

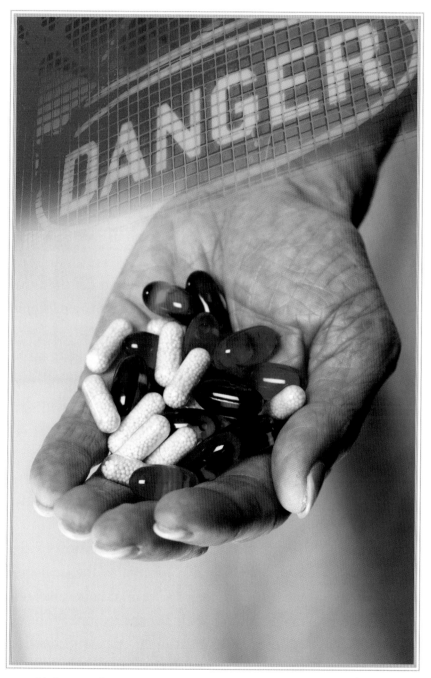

All drug advertisements must contain comprehensive warnings regarding any dangers to consumers.

certainly be how those advertisements affect consumer perceptions of drugs.

When the FDA permitted DTC advertising, it also set down advertising guidelines for the pharmaceutical companies to follow. One of the key measures in those guidelines is the fact that any advertisement must include a comprehensive warning regarding side effects and risks associated with the medicine being advertised. To some extent, this mirrors the concerns over the control of negative information that some companies seem to exercise. The SSRI Paxil provides us with a good illustration of this issue.

In 2001, before the lawsuit brought against GlaxoSmithKline regarding increased suicide risk in young people, people who claimed to have formed addictions to Paxil brought two other lawsuits against the company. Until then, GlaxoSmithKline had maintained that Paxil was non-habit forming, just as all of the other SSRIs appeared to be. Advertisements for Paxil touted that characteristic as a major selling point. In court, however, GlaxoSmithKline's claims did not hold up. The judge in one of the trials forced the company to stop advertising Paxil as non-habit forming. In essence, the company had to admit that Paxil was addictive.

GlaxoSmithKline, however, appealed the decision to the FDA, which then asked the judge to reverse the decision. The FDA argued that the authority to regulate pharmaceutical companies should rest not with the courts, but with the FDA. The judge relented, and reversed the decision, allowing GlaxoSmithKline to continue advertising Paxil as non-habit forming.

Today, the Web site for Paxil still claims that the drug is non-habit forming. It qualifies this statement, however, by adding "you may have symptoms on stopping Paxil." The site then lists some of these symptoms, including headaches, stomach pains, diarrhea, unexplained sweating, tremors, and fatigue. Though GlaxoSmithKline evidently does not consider this a list of withdrawal symptoms, it certainly reads like one.

Lobbying

In recent years, a great deal of pressure has been put on the pharmaceutical industry by federal legislators. The increasing cost of health care has become a sensitive topic for many people throughout North America. In the United States, many—

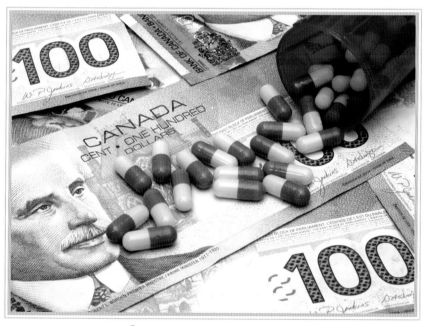

In Canada, the high cost of prescription drugs contributes to high taxes.

particularly the elderly—fear that they will not be able to afford medical care or medicines, and that their insurance will not cover them for many expenses. In Canada, people point to the high cost of health care as one cause of high taxes. In both countries, taxpayers, consumers, and lawmakers alike say that the pharmaceutical companies are profiting at the expense of the people, and that the high cost of health care is creating an undue burden on the economy.

The pharmaceutical industry has not taken these claims idly, though. The Pharmaceutical Research and Manufacturers of America—PhRMA—is an association of many different pharmaceutical companies that have pooled their resources, largely for the purpose of improving the public image of the pharmaceutical industry. In addition, PhRMA uses its resources to provide a variety of social action programs for the benefit of underserved populations. The PhRMA Web site provides information about the prescription drug assistance programs PhRMA offers to patients who might not otherwise be able to receive medications they need. The site also lists the donations to catastrophe relief efforts that member companies make. In the wake of the 2006 Hurricane Katrina disaster in New Orleans, for example, PhRMA members donated nearly 130 million dollars worth of medical supplies to disaster relief agencies and hospitals.

One thing that the Web site does not seem to discuss is the *lobbying* presence of PhRMA and its *constituent* companies. In 1999 and 2000, the pharmaceutical industry spent about 200 million dollars on lobbying efforts and campaign contributions, even more than they spent on Hurricane Katrina relief. Probably not coincidentally, in the past several years, a number of new laws have been passed that stand to benefit pharmaceutical manufacturers. The most well known of these new laws is the Medicare Modernization Act of 2003, which gives senior citizens prescription drug coverage benefits that are paid for through taxpayer money. On the one hand, the law will almost certainly help many elderly people who need access to medicine. On the other hand, the pharmaceutical industry will profit tidily through taxpayers' money.

Conclusion

The example of the Medicare Modernization Act may best summarize the issues surrounding the pharmaceutical industry. The industry does many things that help people live better, longer lives. In this respect, many people apparently owe the industry a debt of gratitude. On the other hand, the industry profits greatly from its position and role, and wields such clout that it would be difficult to rein it in. In this respect it seems we're paying for that debt of gratitude every time we have to buy expensive medicines.

The pharmaceutical industry is a difficult thing to characterize for these reasons and more. Looking at the industry and its activities closely, there may be no real answers as to the right and wrong of it. What do you think?

Further Reading

Cefrey, Holly. *Antidepressants.* New York: Rosen Publishing Group, 2000.

Dudley, W. ed.. *Antidepressants (History of Drugs).* Chicago, Ill.: Greenhaven Press, 2004.

Dunbar, Katherine Read, ed. *Antidepressants.* Detroit, Mich.: Greenhaven Press, 2005.

Esherick, Joan. *Drug Therapy and Anxiety Disorders.* Broomall, Pa.: Mason Crest, 2004.

Esherick, Joan. *Drug Therapy and Mood Disorders.* Broomall, Pa.: Mason Crest, 2004.

Esherick, Joan. *The FDA and Psychiatric Drugs: How a Drug Is Approved.* Broomall, Pa.: Mason Crest, 2004.

Ford, Jean. *Surviving the Roller Coaster: A Teen's Guide to Coping with Moods.* Broomall, Pa.: Mason Crest, 2005.

Keena, Kathleen. *Adolescent Depression: Outside/In.* Lincoln, Neb.: iUniverse, Inc., 2005.

Kim, Henny, ed. *Depression.* San Diego, Calif.: Greenhaven Press, 2000.

Packard, Helen C. *Prozac: The Controversial Cure.* New York: Rosen Publishing Group, 2001.

Wurtzel, Elizabeth. *Prozac Nation: Young and Depressed in America: A Memoir.* New York: Riverhead Books, 1997.

For More Information

Eli Lilly
www.lilly.com

FDA
www.fda.gov

GlaxoSmithKline
us.gsk.com

Paxil
www.paxil.com

PhRMA
www.phrma.org

Prozac
www.prozac.com

SSRIs
www.biopsychiatry.com/ssris.htm

Publisher's note:
The Web sites listed on this page were active at the time of publication. The publisher is not responsible for Web sites that have changed their addresses or discontinued operation since the date of publication. The publisher will review and update the Web-site list upon each reprint.

Glossary

charisma: The ability to inspire enthusiasm, interest, or affection in others by means of personal charm.

constituent: Someone who appoints another to act on his or her behalf.

controversial: Provoking strong disagreements.

derivatives: Things that have developed from something else that are similar to them.

diphtheria: A bacterial disease that attacks the throat and releases a toxin that damages the heart and nervous system.

drug regimens: Strict routines for taking medications.

efficacy: The ability to produce the necessary or desired results.

engendered: Caused something to come into existence.

extracts: Concentrates or purified substances obtained by dissolving this substance with solvent when present with other materials and then evaporating the solvent.

farcical: Resembling a farce in being ridiculous and confused.

icon: A cultural emblem or symbol.

inconclusive: Not producing a clear-cut result.

indiscriminate: Random.

inhumane: Lacking compassion and causing excessive suffering.

innovation: Something new.

lobbying: Representing the interests of those trying to influence political policy.

obsessive-compulsive disorder: A psychiatric disorder characterized by recurring thoughts and the irresistible need to perform certain behaviors.

over-the-counter: Available to the public without a prescription.

potent: Powerful.

poultices: Warm, moist preparations placed on an aching or inflamed part of the body to reduce pain.

regulatory agency: An organization that controls activity and makes certain that rules are complied with.

schizophrenia: A psychiatric disorder characterized by a loss of contact with reality.

sedative: Something that soothes or calms.

seizure: A convulsion.

skepticism: A sense of suspicion or doubt.

stimulant: Something that increases activity levels.

synthesized: Produced a substance by combining elements into a new whole.

tetanus: An infectious disease usually contracted through an open wound, which causes severe muscular spasms and contractions, especially around the neck and jaw.

theatrics: Staged or contrived effects.

tuberculosis: A serious, highly infectious lung disease.

variables: Things capable of changing.

veritable: Indicating that something being referred to figuratively is as good as true.

Bibliography

Antonucci, David O., and William G. Danton. "Psychology in the Prescription Era: Building a Firewall Between Marketing and Science." *American Psychologist* 58, no. 12 (December 2003): 1028–1043.

"Advertised Prescription Drugs Are the Hot Sellers." *Drug Benefit Trends* 14, no. 4 (2002): 4. http://www.medscape.com/viewarticle/432386.

Advertisement for Dr. Chase's Nervous Pills. *Newark Advocate*. Newark, Ohio. December 6, 1904.

Arndt, Michael. "Eli Lilly: Life After Prozac." *Business Week Online*, July 23, 2001. http://www.businessweek.com/magazine/content/01_30/b3742106.htm.

Associated Press. "Lawsuit: Paxil Addictive, has Serious Side Effects." *USA Today*, September 1, 2001. http://www.usatoday.com/news/nation/2001/09/18/paxil-suit.htm.

Associated Press. "Spitzer Sues GlaxoSmithKline over Paxil." MSNBC.com, June 2, 2004. http://www.msnbc.msn.com/id/5120989.

Baker, C. Bruce, Michael T. Johnsrud, M. Lynn Crismon, Robert A. Rosenheck, and Scott W. Woods. "Quantitative Analysis of Sponsorship Bias in Economic Studies of Antidepressants." *British Journal of Psychiatry* 183 (2003): 498–506.

Crellin, John K. *A Social History of Medicines in the Twentieth Century: To Be Taken Three Times a Day.* Binghamton, N.Y.: Pharmaceutical Products Press, 2004.

"From Quackery to Bacteriology: The Emergence of Modern Medicine in the 19th Century." University of Toledo Libraries. http://www.cl.utoledo.edu/canaday/quackery/quack-index.html.

"Glaxo Settles Paxil Lawsuit." CBSNews.com, August 26, 2004. http://www.cbsnews.com/stories/2004/06/03/health/main620815.shtml.

Hawkins, Beth. "Paxil Is Forever." *Minneapolis/St. Paul City Pages* 23, issue 1141 (October 16, 2002). http://www.citypages.com/databank/23/1141/article10788.asp.

Healy, David. *The Antidepressant Era.* Cambridge, Mass.: Harvard University Press, 1999.

Healy, David. *Let Them Eat Prozac: The Unhealthy Relationship Between the Pharmaceutical Industry and Depression.* New York: New York University Press, 2004.

"Is It Prozac? Or Placebo?" http://www.motherjones.com/news/feature/2003/11/ma_565_01.html.

Lipsky, Martin S., and Lisa K. Sharp. "From Idea to Market: The Drug Approval Process." *Journal of the American Board of Family Practice* 14, no. 5 (2001): 362–367.

Mossinghoff, Gerald J. "Overview of the Hatch-Waxman Act and Its Impact on the Drug Development Process." *Food and Drug Law Journal* 54, no. 2 (1999): 187–194.

"North American Pharmaceutical Sales Growth Up 12 Percent; Continues to Lead Major Markets." *IMS World Review 2003*. February 25, 2003.

Rosenheck, Robert. "The Growth of Psychopharmacology in the 1990s: Evidence-Based Practice or Irrational Exuberance." *International Journal of Law and Psychiatry* 28 (2005): 467–483.

"Securities Class Action Lawsuit Against GSK Over Paxil." *PR Newswire*, April 18, 2005. http://www.legalnewswatch.com/news_568.html.

"Suit Filed Against Antidepressant Paxil." CNN.com, August 25, 2001. http://www.antidepressantsfacts.com/CNN_com-classaction-paxil.htm.

Index

Picture Credits

Benjamin Stewart: pp. 70, 76, 86, 90, 97
iStockphotos: pp. 22, 81
    Andrey Nikolajew: p. 78
    Jill Frommer: p. 85
    Martin Bowker: p. 55
    Matt Matthews: p. 24
    Mikhail Tolstoy: p. 39
    Shaun Lowe: p. 99
    Tom McNemar: p. 82
Jupiter Images: pp. 65, 67, 68, 72, 75, 93, 94
National Library of Medicine: pp. 8, 11, 13, 15, 18, 33, 40, 43, 52
U.S. Department of Agriculture: pp. 34, 36, 48, 56, 60, 62
U.S. Food and Drug Administration: pp. 29, 30
U.S. Postal Service: p. 26
World Health Organization: p. 44

Biographies

Author

David Hunter is the author of two other books and several articles published in educational magazines. He came by the topic of pharmaceuticals quite naturally, having grown up around medicine. His father is a hospital pharmacist, and his mother was a nurse. David is himself planning on going back to school for graduate work in nursing.

Consultant

Andrew M. Kleiman, M.D., received a Bachelor of Arts degree in philosophy from the University of Michigan, and earned his medical degree from Tulane University School of Medicine. Dr. Kleiman completed his internship, residency in psychiatry, and fellowship in forensic psychiatry at New York University and Bellevue Hospital. He is currently in private practice in Manhattan, specializing in psychopharmacology, psychotherapy, and forensic psychiatry. He also teaches clinical psychology at the New York University School of Medicine.